You Are
WHY
You Eat

CHANGE YOUR FOOD ATTITUDE,
CHANGE YOUR LIFE

DR. RAMANI DURVASULA

Foreword by Vanessa Williams

Guilford, Connecticut
An imprint of Globe Pequot Press

skirt® is an attitude . . . spirited, independent, outspoken, serious, playful and irreverent, sometimes controversial, always passionate.

Project editor: Ellen Urban
Text design and layout: Maggie Peterson

Library of Congress Cataloging-in-Publication Data

Durvasula, Ramani.
  You are why you eat : change your food attitude, change your life /
Dr. Ramani Durvasula.
     pages cm
  Summary: "An intelligent, timely, and prescriptive book that shows how
your attitude towards food often reflects your attitude towards other
areas in your life—jobs, relationships, money—and how you can let go
of trying to please others all the time and instead satisfy your own
true appetites and live a more authentic and healthier life"— Provided
by publisher.
  ISBN 978-0-7627-8245-1 (hardback)
  1. Food habits—Psychological aspects. 2. Health—Psychological
aspects. I. Title.
  TX357.D84 2013
  394.1'2—dc23
                                                    2012033961

Printed in the United States of America

10 9 8 7 6 5 4 3 2

The material in this book is intended to provide accurate and authoritative information, but should not be used as a substitute for professional care. The author and publisher urge you to consult with your mental health care provider or seek other professional advice in the event that you require expert assistance.

To Maya Sai Hinkin and Shanti Lindeman Hinkin

—MY ANGELS—

who make me brave and let my spider senses sing.

To my muse, William Wallis Pruitt,
for awakening the poet inside of me
and reminding us every day to live the questions.

"If you want the truth,
I'll tell you the truth:
Listen to the secret sound,
the real sound,
which is inside you"
—Kabir

CONTENTS

FOREWORD

Is it ever easy for any of us to listen to ourselves? I know that in my career, I have had times when I didn't listen to myself, and when things went wrong, I knew that if I had listened to myself (and my mother) in the first place, I could have avoided a lot of trouble (Ramani calls these our "spider senses"). I struggled with sorting through the different kinds of advice I got from different kinds of stakeholders. But I learned from these experiences and let them guide me to new paths in the future and a career that I have loved at every turn of the road. At the end of the day, each of us knows what is best for us, but sometimes we need to make a few mistakes to get there. Life is a journey, and Ramani's book is about making an authentic journey that is led by the compass that each of us has within us.

As a woman, especially one who works in the very public business of entertainment, I have lived under the glare of having my body and face scrutinized as long as I could remember. As the mother of daughters of varying ages, and from watching my friends, I know that issues of food, weight, and body image are a burden that women of all ages, races, and kinds struggle with. What is so bold about Ramani's stance is that for once, someone is telling us our bodies are a good thing and when we listen to our bodies, our hearts, and our minds, we are more likely to find a greater balance than just trying the next new diet or depriving ourselves of the foods we enjoy. She and I are foodies. When we eat out together, we comment on the struggles that a bowl of pasta can bring, and she has taught me some interesting tips.

And let's face it, the heart and the stomach are connected in many ways, and Ramani and I have dished a lot about relationships, heartache, and men. It often comes back to the same place—listen to yourself, honor yourself, treat yourself the way you want a partner to treat you—and I love that Ramani is suggesting that you start by doing this at the table. Once you start getting respect for yourself in one area of your life, it will follow in others.

By helping each of us see that this is a journey that is both inside of us but also impacted by the world outside of us, it helps us understand the battles we need to wage inside of us, while we have to live in a complex food world. On one hand the world is telling us to be a size 2, and on the other it is shoving burgers and pie in our faces. This book doesn't deny that reality, and tells us that there is no getting around it; we have to learn to eat in a challenging world, and only we know our own bodies.

I have watched Ramani's journey myself, and we became friends when she was going through a divorce and struggling with listening to herself, so I know that she not only has the scientific and psychological chops behind this but also the personal insight and struggle. She is able to communicate her complex ideas in a simple way that I know will change so many lives. I know her beautiful daughters, Maya and Shanti, and I know her as both a friend and as a mother. She gets it, and she has lived it.

Whether you are looking to change your dress size or your love life, take on your dreams, or just figure out how to connect back to yourself again so you can live a healthy, fulfilled, and authentic life, Ramani's book will take you there. A message lives inside this book for almost everyone I know, and I am confident that Ramani's voice will change your view of the world and open you up to yourself. I'm so glad the world will finally get to read her words.

Vanessa Williams, Chappaqua, NY

INTRODUCTION

The Watts Towers stand tall above a gritty urban neighborhood in South Los Angeles. A man named Sam Rodia, a laborer, not an artist, spent thirty-three years of his life building them between the years of 1921 and 1954.

He found a small triangular lot in his neighborhood and started collecting rebar, scrap salvaged from the railroad, and other found objects that he stacked and welded together. Slowly, the towers began to emerge and take shape. They are a unique tribute to urban art, to a neighborhood rarely visited by most Angelenos, and speak to the dedication of one man. Each time you look at them, new details emerge. They are most certainly a national treasure.

These towers were a massive undertaking, and Rodia built them alone—scaling the ninety-nine feet up with harnesses and climbing the structures like ladders to ensure his work reached greater heights. He was a quirky guy and often found himself in conflict with his neighbors, but he persisted. When asked why he worked so tirelessly on these towers, he simply said, "I wanted to do something big, and I did it."

Even more compelling is the fact that suddenly, one day, he was done. He just finished. There was still more space, more time, and more stuff to stack. But he stopped. He was simply done. In short order he packed up and moved away to Martinez, California, where he lived until his death in 1965.

—◁○▷—

How often do people know they are "done"? How often do they know when to walk away from a project, from a relationship, from a job, from a casino table, from a sale, from a conflict? Well, the simple answer is: not often enough. Hell, most people don't know how to walk away from a plate of food when they are full. A recent CBS news poll found that 54 percent of Americans almost always eat until their plate is clean. And that's the problem. The way we eat has some heavy implications for our lives. Most people think simply cutting carbs or working with a trainer will help them lose weight, but that's not the case. Understanding why you are eating or getting a second helping is a much greater tool than following strict, arbitrary rules written by someone else. It's your body—you should know what it likes. As soon as you can understand the psychology to your eating, you'll lose weight. And the rest of your life will fall into place as well.

That's where *You Are WHY You Eat* comes in. This book is about learning how to quit, when to quit, when to walk away, and how to acknowledge when you are full. It is about trusting yourself and knowing that you are full—even if that means leaving behind a plate full of food. It's about turning off the voices of the world and listening to the one that matters most: your own.

Rodia knew he was done. And after reading this book, you will, too.

Start by asking yourself one simple but significant question: Does your life look the way you want it to look? Has the weight you have put on taken control of everything you do? Does the thought of losing it seem impossible, or overwhelming? Sadly, most of us are living a script written by other people, and as a result of this, many of us learned long ago to stop listening to our own instincts. We don't often trust ourselves. It's easier to do what the world asks of us than to blaze our own trail. If you do what the world wants, then you are a hero; if you do what you want, you are selfish. But when we defy our instincts, our sense of what is right for us, far greater problems can arise. Weight gain is one of the most common.

When I was training to be a psychologist, it became clear that one of the key issues in human growth is taking responsibility. Unfortunately, we have gotten to a place where taking responsibility has become more about apologizing after the fact, rather than weighing out what we want to do and thinking about the ramifications ahead of time. Personally, I'm working harder than I ever have before; the stress of being a divorced mother is enormous, and I have more to juggle and deal with financially and logistically than I ever did when I was married. But I'm incredibly satisfied with my life, and despite the fatigue, financial crises, and uncertainty, my life is characterized by possibility and joy.

Believe me when I say: It wasn't an easy place at which to arrive. I was pretty miserable, in fact. To ease my misery, I turned to food. I over-ate because I was in a dark place in life for a long time. I knew my marriage wasn't working, so I just kept eating. I was stressed about my two children, feeling like I didn't measure up as a mother, so I kept eating. I didn't love my work, so I kept eating. I was lonely, so I kept eating.

Food became a distraction—a place to numb myself, reward myself, and soothe myself. It allowed me to not think about the other stuff. I didn't know how to stop eating when I was full because I was using food to do too many things. I didn't know how to walk away from my plate or how to trust my instincts. So exactly how would I have gone about fixing the big-ticket issues in my life if I couldn't do something as simple as walking away from the table when I was full?

There was literally a moment for me when I knew I had to make some major changes in my life. The problem, though, was that when I took stock of what needed fixing, I realized my marriage and my career were two things that were simply too enormous to take on. The wake-up call came when my youngest daughter, who was two years old at the time, became seriously ill. After a hospitalization and IV medications at home for a month for her, my husband and I had the chance to attend a wedding, our first night out in months. I knew life had gotten the best of me, and that I had put on some weight. I grabbed some oversize garments my mother had brought back from India and figured I would "toss" them on. I had become so big that as I pulled them on, the delicate silks just tore. I went through three dresses and ended up choosing the one that had torn the least.

I knew that I'd gained weight, but had no idea just how much, exactly. If you had asked me to guesstimate, I would have probably thought I weighed around 160 pounds. I popped on the scale, which I hadn't stepped on for about two years, and to my genuine surprise, I topped 200 pounds.

I knew at that moment that *something* had to be done, but I still didn't know what to do, or how to do it. That night at the wedding I ate like it was my last night on Earth. I ate my meal, the entire contents of the breadbasket, and half of my husband's dinner. My husband wanted to get home to our child, but I refused to leave before the cake came out. I was on a mission, and I wasn't leaving until I'd shoveled it all in.

The next day, still stuffed, I went to a farmers' market with my family and I ate burgers—plural. I literally went on a bender. That was September 30, 2005. In some ways, I knew this was it—that I would never eat this way again. I was saying good-bye to a lifestyle.

On October 1, 2005, I vowed never to return. I jumped on the scale and started my journey weighing 201 pounds and wearing a size 18.

I took stock of a life that was a mess, and realized that most of the other changes I needed to make would impact other people. There was my weight, and there was everything else that needed fixing. As for the "everything else"—well, I wasn't ready to take all of that on yet. But food was within my control. My attitude was that if I failed at this weight-loss experiment, then life could go on as it had been. I had no weight-loss goal; I just wanted to see if I could ease up on the food intake and maybe start to exercise (at that time I would get winded after going up a flight of stairs). I knew what I put into my mouth was the one thing I could control at that moment.

I started small. I excavated the treadmill in the corner of the playroom and I started with walking just five minutes a day. I increased my routine by five minutes on weeks I didn't lose any weight. I didn't go to a dietitian or a trainer; I just used basic common sense. I got rid of the junk food in my diet and made a promise to myself that I wouldn't get to the point where I let myself feel hungry (a feeling that often resulted in panic for me). I allowed myself unlimited fruits and vegetables (because no one really ever binges on broccoli). My new food reality was simple: It was no longer ten cookies, it was one. It was no longer a burger and fries. It was chicken and vegetables.

Was this easy? No. Is it easy to this day? Nope—not even close. Is it still a struggle? Would I prefer to eat burgers every day? Absolutely. Did I need to lock the cupboards in the kitchen and pour soap on leftovers so I didn't eat them? Yes. But I lost ten pounds in six weeks, and by the time I'd lost twelve pounds, people started to notice, and that gave me the strength to keep at it. Ten pounds became eighty-five pounds, and the original five minutes on the treadmill became an hour a day, and eventually hiking mountains around the world.

There was an extra reward to shedding that weight: I gained another kind of strength along the way. As I started losing the weight, I felt able to make other, bigger, more life-altering decisions. It was like my spider senses—the term I use to describe those true gut feelings we use to guide us—were numbed by the weight, and once I was able to get the weight off, my senses were sharper. I also believed in my power and ability to make a change. Knowing we need to change something is only half the battle in life; actually making the change is the payoff. The weight loss created an awareness that made me realize, yes, my marriage wasn't working, and I could fix that situation too by applying the same techniques.

With a stronger mind, body, and heart, I started being able to heed my instincts when it came to the big-ticket items in my life. I was able to have painful conversations with my husband, which had seemed unthinkable years before. I made career changes and forays into the media space, despite professional resistance by my academic world.

There was an extra reward to shedding that weight. I gained another kind of strength along the way.

Throughout the process, which was arduous, I felt the disapproving voices of those around me. Friends, parents, in-laws, and colleagues called me out on it, saying, "You don't know what you're doing. . . . You're making a huge mistake. . . . You're going to regret all of this for the rest of your life. . . . You are destroying your children; they will be from a broken home." But I inherently knew that what I was doing felt right. I felt like I was at the edge of a cliff and that I was going to jump, but with a parachute on my back. Everyone around me told me that the parachute would not open, but the chute was really just trusting myself, and I fully intended to take the leap. I closed my ears to the advice from the people around me. I came to realize that they were terrified because my choices impacted them. My actions would not only call their own actions into question, but would also change their lives. I jumped.

The chute opened.

I am now a happily divorced woman. I consider my ex-husband to be one of my closest friends. We regularly spend time together with our children and have moved on with our lives. We have constructed a new kind of family, one that really works. The weight is still off and my body is stronger than ever.

THE DARK SIDE OF LISTENING TO YOU

It was risky. I had to make a choice, and there were downsides; I could either stay the course and honor myself, or stay in a life that felt wrong.

Some people tried to coax me back to my eating days to draw me back to being the person I once was. (When someone puts sweets and dessert in front of me, I still feel like an alcoholic in recovery.) Some continue to label me selfish—a villain, a sellout, and a family wrecker. That is the hard part about honoring your instincts; it means making enormous changes, and before it became easy for me, I knew it was going to become very hard. But the discovery that came from the weight loss was that it is okay to leave food on my plate when I know I am full; it is okay to listen to myself. It is okay to start taking care of me.

Sounds simple, doesn't it? When I look back, I wonder why I didn't take back my life sooner, before I turned forty. But looking backwards is generally a waste of time. I learned to honor myself on my time, and my life has been spectacular ever since. Easier? No. More authentic? Yes. I do realize now that the main thing that held me back was my fear of the body count, of disappointing people, of losing people. The fear of losing people who would be, were, and are affected by my choices. I made some real sacrifices to live a real life.

As you read *You Are WHY You Eat,* these consequences will be addressed in a real way. There is a body count and collateral damage when you honor your instincts. Family members told me that when I got married and had children, I should give up on my dreams. Many family members rejected me entirely for my decisions, and while some have since come around, I have lost contact with several of my family members. I defied the rules of order in my family and my culture, and it cost me.

A NEW LIFE RISING FROM THE ASHES

The holes left by the losses have been sumptuously filled—by exquisite friends, happy children, a wonderful career, and a great love. As we honor our spider senses, which you'll read about more comprehensively throughout this book, and learn to listen to ourselves, we become more skilled at knowing what and whom to let in (or out), and how we spend our time. The naysayers from my old life aren't in my life anymore, and my social and family landscape looks very different today than it did back in the old days. The people who populate my world now are different stakeholders; they celebrate my successes and console me when I fail, but most important, they revel in the fact that I honor my spider senses, while I do the same for them. By becoming more authentic, the people who enter my life are also more authentic.

Many times, denying our own spider senses—our inner voice, our sense of being "in tune" with ourselves—can yield a smaller body count, but at a great cost to ourselves. There's a great analogy in war: A soldier jumps on a grenade to save his team; one dies so many others can live. There is a certain perceived nobility in that. Many people stay in bad relationships and marriages, unsatisfying jobs, and unfulfilling lives so they can "save" the people around them. Life is not a grenade, and trying to avoid the disappointment of others is not about heroism but often about fear. If we can learn that while initially there will be loss and pain, in the long term, the hurts will heal, and even those who were hurt by you honoring yourself may be propelled into a more honest life. In addition, the example you set by honoring yourself, and doing so without fear, may in the long term enhance many more lives.

Staying in bad situations can cause collateral damage as well. In the short term, staying in a bad situation is easier, despite the long-term damage. But sometimes short-term losses are needed for long-term gains. Do you really think a spouse or intimate partner in a loveless relationship benefits from the disillusioned partner sticking around? Do your children benefit by you sticking it out in an uninspired job? Do you benefit from eating everything on your plate? This book will help you to rewrite your scripts and redefine what makes a hero. It surprised me to learn that honoring my spider senses and simply eating differently led to changes in every arena of my life.

For me, giving up on my dreams and not honoring the life I desired would have ultimately made everyone's lives worse. Heeding my inner compass allowed me to create a new life and a new world. Now, every morning when I wake up, I'm filled with a sense of possibility rather than a sense of despair.

I have stories from patients who weren't so lucky—examples of people who lost more by staying in something bad rather than accepting that they were "full," and leaving, or quitting. Many of these people have reached the latter part of life filled with regrets, but are now realizing that it's not too late to make a change, to honor their instincts. It is likely that my sticking it out and eating everything on my plate would have resulted in far worse outcomes for my children and my health in the long term.

While I definitely made my life more difficult by leaving in a practical sense (financial challenges, single parenthood), I made it authentically better—substantially, tremendously better. Every morning feels like a holiday, every day piled up with potential.

We *can* find peace in chaos. The illusion is that financial comfort, stability, monogamy, and permanence are guarantees of safety and security. After reading this book, you will realize that by honoring yourself and listening to your own inner voice (while managing the voices around you), true security can be found within yourself—even in the midst of day-to-day challenges.

There were lots of wonderful bonuses that occurred when I changed my life. I got bold. I started exploring the world alone, taking trips, and began commemorating each anniversary of my weight loss with a hike. I've climbed to the top of Mount Fuji and been to Mount Everest's base camp, among many others. These were trips I talked myself out of in earlier years—too much money, too much time, I wasn't strong enough. Once I started listening to me, somehow the details came together, the money worked itself out, and I came back a better version of me. The only way you can achieve a successful summit is by honoring your instincts, knowing the best path, knowing when to rest, and knowing when to turn back.

A BETTER LIFE THROUGH BETTER CHOICES AND BETTER VOICES

And that's what this book is about. It's about achieving the most out of life. It's about understanding your needs and trusting yourself. It's about collecting data through experience so you can best assess and execute major decisions in your life. It's about knowing when to stay and when to walk away. It's about making better choices in the beginning, because getting out is a lot harder than getting in, in the first place. It's about balancing the voices in your life with the voice you want to live. It's about food as the metaphor for so many other elements in your life. It's about how to fill your plate, knowing when you are full, and ignoring childhood teachings and golden rules that are based on obedience rather than growth. And if the only thing you learn from *You Are WHY You Eat* is *how* to eat, then you are still ahead of most people who are banging their heads against the dieting wall every day.

I have so many patients who come to see me to discuss their weight, who then realize that this isn't about food or calories or exercise. It's about something bigger in their lives, like loneliness, hurts from the past, lack of intimacy, and damaged scripts that underlie the overeating, disordered eating, and unhealthy eating. Overfull plates are often substitutes for something that just isn't right—for families and other stakeholders that didn't listen, but insisted on clean plates and no questions.

RECORDING YOUR STORY

Ignore the rules you were taught and change things. Be true to you—you know your needs better than anyone does. Are you sure you are full? Even the best-intentioned among us ask that question of our eating companions. Often it is just good manners. But the only way you can answer that question is to be completely honest with yourself. *Are you full?* In this book I'll share stories with you that my patients, associates, friends, family, and colleagues have shared with me. I'll share inspiring quotes and my own life's experience. I'll ask you to do some homework, too, in the form of exercises, which will be offered in every chapter. I'm going to ask you to get a journal, make notes, and really think about the exercises you're going to be asked to complete. A journal can be a blank book, a smartphone, a laptop, or a tablet. It is best if you keep all of this in one place, so you can see the accumulation of the information and watch your own development unfold. I think the best way to tackle this book is to read it at your own pace, and then focus on one chapter a week, and really spend time that week on the exercises in that chapter. For more tips, be sure to check out the *You Are WHY You Eat* app on your smartphone.

Trust yourself. Don't be afraid to try. Don't be afraid to experience. Don't feel you have to stick everything out. When you finish this book, you'll have helped yourself. You'll learn to trust your gut so you won't overfill your gut anymore

This book is your place to express and think and process. It is meant to give you a framework, but more important, it is meant to give you permission—permission to leave food on your plate, to break the rules, to listen to yourself. Use your journal to take notes and complete the exercises I'm going to ask you to dedicate yourself to throughout the chapters. Write everything in this journal.

The clever French writer François Duc de La Rochefoucauld writes, "We are so accustomed to disguising ourselves to others that in the end we become disguised to ourselves." *You Are WHY You Eat* teaches you how to stop disguising yourself—at the dinner table, with your partner, with your family, with your children, at your workplace. Listen to your gut; it's trying to tell you something. In the pages that follow, I will remind you how to do something that you were born knowing how to do. And it will start, and perhaps end, with food.

At the end of each chapter of the book, I will present you with a *why* and a *now*. The Why will summarize the key elements of the chapter, and The Now will provide exercises to make the book actionable and link back to your life today.

THE WHY

I've been where you are. I've struggled, too. And I found that only by being true to me was I able to get to where I am today. Trust yourself, honor yourself. And I want you to know, this is coming not only from my personal weight-loss journey, but also from twenty years of reading, writing, researching, and conducting clinical work. It's also from my experience as a student and a teacher, a patient and a therapist, from being a wife, an ex-wife, a partner, a mother, a sister, a daughter, and a friend.

THE NOW

While I may be the one sharing my story here, it's a universal one. I marked the moment, the very day I changed my life. I said good-bye to an old lifestyle and hello to a new one, and I want you to do the same right now. *You Are WHY You Eat* will teach you how to do this by teaching you how to listen to you.

Your first exercise is to write the new you a letter, and to create your own moment or date to say good-bye to the lifestyle you're about to change. No time like the present! Here's a letter from someone I worked with who was ready to make a change, but feel free to create your own, with your preferred style or way of writing.

Dear Future Me:

I'm writing to let you know that the old me is saying
good-bye to a lot of things. Today, this 26th of January,
I'm saying good-bye to eating when I'm not hungry, being
the person all of my friends call on when they want a
partner in crime to overindulge with, and to the weight
that has accompanied my overly easygoing self. The new
me is ordering what I want to eat at dinner out, not what
everyone else wants to split. I've spent a lifetime being
accommodating—I go with the flow and I really never mind
letting someone else choose a restaurant or a movie. But I
have found, as a result, that I never stand up for myself with
food either. I'm not blaming others for how I eat or how
I got here, but today, I'm speaking up for myself, starting
now. If I don't want to start dinner with deep-fried calamari,
then I'm going to say so instead of just saying, "Okay." I
think I'll be better able to articulate other things in life that
I want for myself once I can start speaking up about the
little things, too. Then, I want to at least start thinking about
going back to school, making the career shift to get out of
this rut, and start taking some more chances. Just not sure
how to get there yet. . . .

Signed,
The old me

Take out your journal and say good-bye to your old lifestyle and hello
to the new one.

PART ONE:

The WHY Foundation

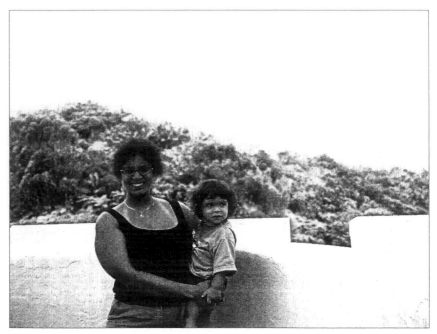

A picture of me and my daughter seven years ago, before I lost 85 pounds and changed my life.

CHAPTER 1

Tapping Your Spider Senses

At the center of your being you have the answer; you know who you are and you know what you want.

—Lao Tzu

There is one premise you should accept as you read this book: *You are the expert of you.* You need to trust yourself in order to find freedom and achieve your destiny. You will learn how this book can be used and how we gain trust in ourselves. You will learn what "being full" means, not just with regard to food, but also in life. This book can be a workbook, it can be a good read, it can be the foundation for a journal; it is a tool to help you unlock a new kind of life.

Do the right thing.

What is the right thing? And what if it's not right for you but is right for someone else in your life?

The writer Henry Miller once wrote, "We slaughter our finest impulses every day," because early in life we learn to live for others. In many cases, our parents want what they think is best for us, as do other family members, friends, and teachers. But what about *you?* What do *you* want for you? And if you listed out what you wanted for yourself, how many of those things are honestly things you want for yourself, and how many of them are you channeling from what the world wants for you?

This chapter will teach you the most important element of this entire book—the foundation on which it's based: learning to tap into and use your spider senses. The term *spider sense* actually originates from the world of Marvel Comics hero, Spider-Man. After Peter Parker endures a bite from a radioactive spider, he gets all kinds of superhuman powers, including the *spider sense*—a sort of sixth sense that allows him to detect danger before it occurs. This allows him to be tuned in and to eliminate any danger before it harms him. Grabbing a rapidly whizzing fly is no small task if you are hanging out in a web, but if you can sense something before it happens, then you are at an advantage, just like a waiting spider.

Thus, a spider sense is a gut instinct, a sense of knowing danger, but also knowing yourself. Spider senses are about the impeccable timing we could all have if we were able to lie as quietly as a spider in a web and listen to ourselves. In *You Are WHY You Eat,* you will have a chance to awaken the spider senses you already have, hopefully without enduring the bite of a radioactive spider.

EVER JUST HAD A FEELING? THOSE ARE YOUR SPIDER SENSES

It's those hairs that stand up on the back of your neck; it's the flutter in your gut, that inherent sense that you know what you need to do—even when it flies in the face of what everyone else wants you to do. You just know. A spider sense is a psychological gut punch. It's a primitive and personal sense of feeling and knowing what to do. It's that reptilian brain that knows something is coming before you can ever see it. It's knowing you.

You use your spider senses every day, and more times than you know for some big-ticket decisions. I can all but guarantee that when you really, truly trusted your spider senses, you made some of the finest, most honest, though perhaps riskiest decisions of your life. Here are some examples of our spider senses in action:

- It's pushing away a half-full plate of food when you are full.
- It's not wanting to go on that second date.
- It's thinking that the smaller college is a better fit for you than the bigger (albeit more prestigious) university.
- It's turning down what seems like a dream job after an unsettling meeting with your potential supervisor.

- It's canceling the wedding a month before the date because it just doesn't feel right.

- It's checking in with your teenage daughter who seems a little off today.

LEARNING TO TAP INTO YOUR SPIDER SENSES AND TUNE OUT THE REST

Every decision we make—every choice, every behavior—is motivated by multiple factors. In fact, when you realize all the things that impact your choices, they don't look like your choices anymore. At the most basic level, biological factors like hunger, thirst, and simple physical needs can drive the choices we make (if we are hungry, we eat). But things start to get complicated when we start factoring in the rest of it. This diagram shows the stuff that circles and impacts your decisions.

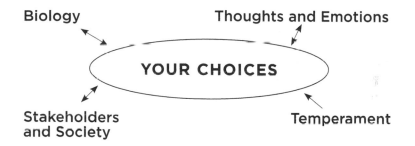

What often gets lost here is what we want, need, and inherently know about ourselves. Our choices and spider senses are not just about biological needs; they are also about us knowing ourselves. They are about a lifetime of accumulated data, of our personalities, of the things we are interested in, of the way we want our lives to look. Think about a person who has driven the same car for a while, or captained the same boat. They know the nuances of how to accelerate, how the vehicle turns, what the little noises and engine pings mean. The same thing applies to us. We know what the little noises and pings mean, but we rarely honor them.

The tricky part of really using our spider senses and making choices is being aware of the things that impact them (the outside elements in the diagram).

Society and Stakeholders

These are the people who are a part of our lives—our moms and dads, boyfriends or husbands, girlfriends or wives. They are our children, our bosses, our friends, and our neighbors. It is all of the childhood teachings and outside forces. Things like our communities, advertisers, and marketers that tell us how to live our lives and spend our money. They can have a huge influence on our choices even if we don't realize it. At the table, this can simply be someone else criticizing us for not eating all of the food on our plate.

Many of my patients can point to one moment when their body image—and subsequently, their relationship with food—shifted. It was usually because of a comment from a stakeholder or a negative experience in their own little society or community, such as in dance class or gymnastics. This moment is pivotal because it's also when they stopped listening to their spider senses.

Thoughts and Emotions

We can talk ourselves into or out of anything. Sometimes we know exactly what we want to do or what we should do, but we think our way *out* of doing it. We rationalize, justify, and compromise with thoughts that are governed by our histories and the world around us. Emotions can be even more powerful, especially our dark emotions, such as depression and anxiety. Any type of mental illness can have a detrimental effect on our spider senses—it causes them to deteriorate and leads to a lot of second-guessing. A typical part of the diagnostic picture of depression, anxiety, and many other mental disorders is self-doubt and feelings of worthlessness. This doubt can definitely scramble spider senses, and sometimes even when someone is not experiencing major depression but just "the blues," self-doubt and second-guessing can really numb your spider senses. Relying on your spider senses means valuing yourself, which is harder to do when you are experiencing sadness or worry.

As a reminder, if you are struggling with chronic feelings of doubt, emptiness, second-guessing, worry, or sadness, I strongly encourage you to talk with your health-care practitioner or a licensed mental health professional.

Stress can also impact these emotions and emotional responses. The biggest scrambler of spider senses is fear. Unless a tiger is chasing you, decisions made on the basis of fear tend to be destructive. Other emotional executioners include envy, greed, doubt, and good, old-fashioned ego. At the table, thoughts and emotions can lead us to eat for reasons unrelated to food—to soothe an emotion, or because we have distorted thoughts about food.

Biology

We all have biological drives over which we have less control. We are driven by hunger and thirst, we have a sex drive, we feel fear in our guts. Our biological drives may lead us to eat, but in general our biology does let us know when we are getting full. And when it comes to complex and emotional decisions such as ending a relationship or leaving a job, biological drives may be of limited utility. Societal norms prevent us from simply responding to our biological drive without some conformity (you don't grab the bread off of your boss's plate at a business lunch because you are hungry). So biology is tempered by reality. At the table, biology is often our friend, and if we just slow down, we can give ourselves the chance to know we are full. But our brains love rewarding food, and once the dopamine starts flowing, sometimes the rewarding taste of that cupcake can override our spider senses that are telling us we have had enough.

Temperament

This is also sometimes termed our personality. A good part of this is inborn; we are born with certain quirks and edges, some of which get smoothed down with time, and some of which are simply who we are. Some of us are risk-takers, some are more open, some are more conscientious—and these temperamental styles will have an impact on how our spider senses are formed, and how we act on what we want. At the table, certain temperamental or personality styles may lead us to feel more compelled to finish everything or to second-guess ourselves.

So what impact do these elements have on your life? Well, these outside forces are like interference that jams up a cell-phone signal. Your instinctual signals, your spider senses, may be clear and clean, but the interference of society and stakeholders can jam up the signal and the spider senses get lost. In life, you often know exactly what you want or need to do, but then, *bam*—the voice of a parent, the disapproval of a friend, or an advertiser that tells you the way your life should look scrambles your signals. For example, you know you want to move to Miami after you graduate, but your mother and father tell you how great your life would be if you stayed in your hometown—that you'd have more friends and a support system, and it's "what you know." Perhaps while you were away at school you knew the best thing for you was to move to Miami. You had it all worked out. Then *bam*—you tell your stakeholders, and they influence your decision. Your signals are scrambled and your decision-making ability impaired.

The only constant in this equation is you. To trust yourself, you need to know what you want, to know that you are full.

The world doesn't know what you want or need; only you do. And much like a waiter in a restaurant does not know if you have had enough to eat and offers you more food for his own purposes, the world offers you advice for its own purposes. The only constant in this equation is you. To trust yourself, you need to know what you want, to know that you are full.

That's where the spider senses come in.

LISTEN TO YOUR GUT—IT'S TELLING YOU SOMETHING

Spider senses have been termed variously in psychological literature as intuitions, hunches, and gut feelings. They get termed "gut instincts" because that's where we feel them. Someone close to me once said, "If your stomach ain't churning, then you ain't learning." There is more than a little truth to that. The fact is, the "gut," as astutely pointed out by researcher Michael Gershon in *The Second Brain,* is populated by nerve cells, and also sitting near that gut are neuroendocrine systems such as the adrenergic system that underlie our "fight or flight" response. All of those tickles in our gut are fast-tracked to the brain, where the decision-making gets executed. So our guts and our brains are soul mates of a sort.

SPIDER SENSES AND DECISIONS

These spider senses, our gut reactions, make us efficient and better—they are a sort of mental and emotional sweet spot. When we follow them, we become efficient because we can make good decisions quickly. Otherwise, every decision we make has to become a new experience. For example, let's look at it through a simple decision: choosing cereal. Over many years of cereal-eating experience, you've established a clear preference. You know what you like. Perhaps you like granola; it's your favorite breakfast cereal. When you walk into the grocery store, if you didn't already know after years of tasting that you like the taste, texture, crunch, and price-point of granola, you'd have to stand in the giant cereal aisle, facing a wall of choices. You'd have to start from scratch to choose something for breakfast, with no data to help you be efficient. But since you know you love granola, you can go directly to the granola section and not be overwhelmed. You don't even have to think about it—you just do it.

Food choices can be complex whether you're in a grocery store, restaurant, or your kitchen at home. The seemingly simple decision about whether to eat a turkey sandwich actually reflects numerous factors, including taste preferences, cravings, beliefs about the food, associations to the food, cost of the food, and then, once we have it, how to eat it (for example, what to put on it), and when to stop eating it. Every sub-choice that feeds into the big choice of acquiring and eating a turkey sandwich is based on our past, present, and future. Yikes! But often our spider senses can quickly lead us to making healthy decisions, as long as we honor them.

Where our spider senses about food can often get thrown is when food has "surplus" meaning. For example, a dessert that feels like a "gift" after a hard day, or a hamburger that is a distraction from the anguish over a broken heart. Food needs to be treated with the mindfulness it deserves. For a moment, think of food as sex. Good sex requires being in the moment, enjoying every taste, smell, and sensation. You don't read a book while having sex (I hope). If, in fact, you are thinking about your taxes or a school project while in the heat of it, you will be distracted and detached (or you may need to rethink how or with whom you are having sex). Sex isn't satisfying if you are having sex to please your partner. In general, we know we should be present while making love, and our spider senses are able to run the show.

It's the same with food. By being present with food—as present as we are during good sex—we listen to our bodies. We chew more slowly and stop when we are full, because we are paying attention to what our bodies are telling us. Perhaps with sex the orgasm lets us know we are done with the main event (and keep in mind that one of the things that can hold us back from orgasm is fear and anxiety—just like knowing whether we are full at the table). It's a shame there isn't a "food orgasm" to tell us when we are done. Don't worry—in this book, I will help you find your food orgasm.

Now let's apply some of what we just discussed about food and spider senses to a grander issue, like dating. You've experienced dating over the years, and you have gained some insight into what works for you and what doesn't. So you go on a first date with a guy and you make some decisions. He lives on the opposite end of town and you say to yourself, "That won't bother me." But he also goes to his mother's house every night for dinner, which you know you can't live with, from past experience. You like hiking, he likes reading, but you know from previous boyfriends that your life is full, and therefore, "I can live without shared interests." What you have is data and experience to help you decide on a second date. It makes it easier to be efficient in deciding, and efficiency brings confidence; therefore, you are making better decisions based on the elegant dance between spider senses and the accumulation of evidence.

Researchers such as Antoine Bechara and Hanna and Antonio Damasio have examined what happens when damage to certain parts of the brain impair connections between emotion and decision-making. The short answer is, it's not good. Our best decisions bring together memory, emotion, intuition, and experience. The brain-damaged patients of Bechara and the Damasios became inefficient at making even basic decisions, largely because they could not benefit from their own experience.

While instincts plus experience can often lead to some efficient and good decisions, there are some factors out there that can really ruin our decisions—things like fear, ego, and revenge. For example, you don't take a new job that might pay less but will have a great career trajectory and might be more rewarding because you're terrified to leave something safe, are worried that you won't be able to cut back on expenses in the short term, or because your spouse/partner is unwilling to bring in more income and you feel responsible as a provider. The same goes for ego or revenge, or letting the world override our spider senses. That's when we do what Mom wants rather than what we want. Not only can we lose efficiency, but we can also make decisions that are not in our best interest when we let these dark clouds impact us. And with that, there's a danger that we'll make a decision that will result in the most catastrophic side effect: regret.

That's why the big-ticket stuff is best done with the use of our spider senses. Buying a home is a great example of this. Research shows that consumer satisfaction is higher when people decide with their gut which house to buy. Don't get me wrong: A home is a big investment, and you need to use a dose of prudence and more than a dash of data in your decision-making recipe, but your spider senses are often most useful when making emotionally laden issues such as purchasing a home and choosing a mate. Freud said it best when he noted: "When making a decision of minor importance, I have always found it advantageous to consider all the pros and cons. In vital matters, however, such as the choice of a mate or a profession, the decision should come from the unconscious, from somewhere within ourselves. In the important decisions of personal life, we should be governed, I think, by the deep inner needs of our nature."

Just as they are built from multiple influences, spider senses are also constantly affected by numerous influences that surround our minds, and us. These factors create the chronic fight between what we know is right and what the world is telling us.

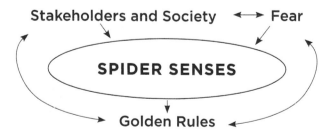

Spider senses are a balancing act—a balance between what we feel and what we already know. Our spider senses serve us best when we are doing something we are familiar with. We know what we want our house to look like, what we want our future partner or spouse to look like, what we want our lives to look like. But this knowing can also be led by scripts rather than by listening to ourselves. Be careful that you are not living a script, because scripts tend to be written by other people, and these scripts tend to be dictated by society. Society is the very thing we as a species created to make our lives better but that has become our worst enemy and is the main blockade to us listening to ourselves. Freud outlined this in his classic work *Civilization and Its Discontents* when he said "it is impossible to overlook the extent to which civilization is built up upon a renunciation of instinct." Simply put, society at some level needs us to silence our spider senses. Freud argued that this disconnect between spider senses and society is a primary source of our unhappiness or discontent. Always remember that you are free to make the choice between what you want and what society wants for you. After reading this book, I hope you will be more willing to tell society to take a powder and start listening to yourself. Applying spider senses when faced with the unknown or in new life experiences can be difficult, but in the absence of data, spider senses are a great place to start.

In order to really grasp the essence of *You Are WHY You Eat,* you need to be able to reconnect to those spider senses and trust them. You need to find your personal minefields and consider them when making decisions, because they often blow up and jam our spider senses.

We will start the journey into your spider senses at the first place you learned to deny them: the dinner table. How many babies keep getting fed when they are already full? How many times were you told to finish everything on an overfull plate? You know when you're full, but you keep picking anyway. You eat when you're not hungry. You refuse to throw away food. Your spider senses tell you that you are full, but lots of things unrelated to food keep you eating. Trusting our spider senses is the backbone of *You Are WHY You Eat.* It's about using data and your own intuition to make a decision, and making honest decisions by honoring yourself instead of the loud voices around you.

THE WHY

Remember to tune in to your spider senses today and in the coming days. Really think about your instinct to do one thing over another, even with tiny decisions you make. Be aware of your initial feeling on something you're deciding, like what to wear when you wake up in the morning or what you eat during mealtime. Start with the smallest things, and eventually you'll learn how to pay attention to your spider senses with the bigger-ticket items, too.

Remember: Your spider senses are your instincts, and it's time to invite them into everything you do. If you want to really embrace and experience the benefits of *You Are WHY You Eat,* I encourage you to do the exercises you'll find in each chapter and record them in your journal. Set aside a few minutes after you read each chapter and give them a try. You might find that some of them will become a part of your daily routine.

THE NOW

One of the simplest experiments I can think of for you to try is to eat plainly. No TV. No book. Not in the car. Not standing up, but seated comfortably, and present. Listen to your body as you chew. Here's the key: Stop when you are full. Try this: Leave your desk when you have lunch, even if it's just for ten minutes. If possible, sit at your table at home and just eat. This kind of mindfulness takes back the control and allows you a greater breadth of choices. At a restaurant, don't order the salad you don't really want simply because it feels virtuous; instead, order the sandwich you *do* want and eat a smaller portion, because you know you can listen to your body and stop when you're full.

By letting your spider senses lead the way, you are more likely to eat what you want, when you want, and as much as you need, rather than eating what a diet book tells you, at the time it prescribes, and finishing a plate of food without thinking or having "cheat days" when you feel out of control after a week of deprivation. Make love to that plate and *be* with it. Document how it felt when you were full, and how the experiences are different than eating food on the go, or while doing something else.

———◦———

Now let's apply this philosophy to your life on a broader scale. In this exercise you are to start by thinking about some big- (and perhaps some not-so-big-) ticket decisions from your life.

Make a list of three decisions in your life where you really trusted your gut instincts. This could be a job, a car, a vacation, a relationship, or even something that other people thought was crazy.

Make a list of three decisions in your life where you deliberately ignored your gut and honored the advice of others over your own wants and needs. Did you ever listen to your father about taking a job that you knew didn't feel right? Have you ever listened to a friend who told you to stop dating a good guy with no money, or to your mother who convinced you not to study abroad because she thought you should save money instead?

Using a scale of 1 to 10, where 10 is perfect and 1 is a failure, rate how each of these decisions ended up working out for you in the long run.

Look at the patterns in terms of outcomes—were the scores higher when you listened to your gut or when you did not?

This is an exercise you can keep adding to as you go through the book; you are likely to recall more and more experiences when you did (and did not) listen to your spider senses. Write them down; they will be valuable data.

WEEKLY CHECK-IN EXERCISE

Throughout the book we will have a "check-in" exercise—something designed to be done every day (if you want to). It allows you to become more mindful about how to connect the concepts from *You Are WHY You Eat* with your daily life, and help you to make sustainable changes that can lead you to a better life in every realm of your world.

CHECK-IN: SPIDER SENSES

It sometimes helps to realize that you are already doing what you need to do. At the end of each day, or at some set time when you have a moment (waiting in line to pick up your kids, before bedtime, when you brush your teeth), think about a situation during the day when you honored your spider senses and made a decision based on intuition and knowing yourself. Some examples could include: throwing away the second half of your sandwich because you're full, saying no to something at work, sharing honest feelings with a partner. It's not the behavior that's important; what's important is that you choose something that you did from a "spider-sense-y place." It may have been doing something that would be counterintuitive to the world: for example, canceling a lunch date because the person makes you feel uncomfortable, or leaving behind a big plate of food instead of taking home the leftovers. When you do this, think about what led you to behave the way you did, how it felt, and if it went against what others wanted. Then reflect on this: Why were you able to ignore those forces?

Over the course of several days and weeks of doing this, I'm going to ask you to look for patterns. Do most of your daily examples occur at your workplace, and not at home? It may be that your spider senses function better at work, but not when you're at lunch or with your partner. This is a chance to reflect on aspects of your life where you need to try harder to become more aligned with *you,* and other places where you see the decision-making process in your life actually working. It's good to be reminded that it does work.

CHAPTER 2

Stakeholders and Their Hold on You

Care about what other people think and you will always be their prisoner.

—Lao Tzu

Whether you're a strong-willed person, a wallflower, a follower, or a trail-blazer, we all have what I call stakeholders in our lives: people whose lives are influenced by you and who influence your life. They might have something to gain by a decision you've made, or they might have something to lose if you choose a different route. They might guide you gently or impact your decisions with an iron fist. Either way, they are a big part of your life.

Who is a stakeholder in your life? The typical short list: your mom, your dad, your spouse or partner, your best friend, your coworker, and your neighbor. But in reality, anyone who is affected by your choices and cares about what happens to you is a stakeholder.

STAKEHOLDERS

Mothers	Coworkers
Fathers	Neighbors
Brothers and sisters	Employers
Partners and spouses	Extended family
Children	Strangers
Friends	

Many times, these stakeholders have their own agendas. Some people's husbands want them to stay overweight. Mothers want their daughters to keep eating their lasagna because it makes them feel good about their cooking. Some people around you may be rooting for your weight loss, but at the end of the day, they don't want it to throw off their own rhythms, wants, or desires. "Go ahead, lose weight—but tonight, we're eating burgers, so don't interrupt my dinner with your new eating habits." They may not say that outright, but they say it subtly, or in a way that makes you feel guilty.

Stakeholders contribute to how we eat, love, work, and live. Our parents were instrumental in our eating scripts, and the pressure our stakeholders apply doesn't end at the table, or in childhood. The big lesson to remember here: Tuning out your stakeholders at the table can also help you tune them out in life's bigger decisions.

Food was an important way of communicating in my family—a way of exercising control, learning discipline, and communicating love. The power of stakeholders and food became apparent to me recently during a visit home in an attempt to mend fences with my parents. I am careful about what I eat and heed my spider senses whenever possible. However, there I stood while cake was being passed around—a grown woman, completely autonomous from my family. Sweets have always been a challenge for me, so I typically avoid them, and at that moment, at my parents' place, I didn't want them.

My father said, "Show us you love us and eat some of our cake." The adult woman in me was able to say, "No, thank you, I don't want it," which was met with frustration from my father, which made me feel guilty. As I reflected on what he said, I realized there was no way the child in me could have fought that request all those years ago. The contributions of stakeholders to not only my lifelong struggle with weight, but also with many other mistakes I have made, became painfully clear. When you eat, live, love, or work for somebody else, you lose sight of what you need and want. In my case, it resulted in a lifelong struggle not only with weight, but also with living to please others, and subsequently, a lot of bad decisions.

This chapter will identify your stakeholders—the people who are affected by what you do, and what you choose. Keep in mind that these stakeholders are noisy people; they are the Greek chorus of our lives. They are the ones who often fill our plates and then demand that we finish everything on them in order to serve their purposes and agendas. They are generally going to offer advice that brings the least disruption to their lives and validates their choices. But the new, self-aware you is going to learn to balance the voices of your stakeholders against your spider senses.

> *Ignoring your stakeholders at the table can help you ignore them in life's bigger decisions.*

BEWARE OF BLIND OBEDIENCE

In the 1960s, Stanley Milgram, a professor at Yale, was trying to understand why people behave the way they do, especially those who engage in cruel or even evil behavior. He did a series of unforgettable experiments with research volunteers in his lab. Very simply, they were brought into a room in which there was a one-way mirror; through that mirror they could see into another room, where a person was hooked up to a variety of electrodes. A research assistant sat with the volunteer and told him or her that the person on the other side was hooked up to electrodes that would administer a small shock. The research assistant then asked the volunteer to press the button that would administer the shock. Initially, the shocks were not painful, and the person on the other side would sit there and perhaps react mildly to the shock. But then the research assistant told the volunteer to increase the intensity of the shock by turning a dial. It was clear by the reactions of the person on the other side of the glass that these shocks were painful. The volunteers were told that at a certain level, the shocks could seriously harm the person on the other side of the glass, and yet, in nearly 70 percent of cases, the volunteers administered the fullest level of shock because they were told to do so by the research assistant. A person they had never met was telling them to harm another person they had never met. They were obeying the orders of the one who told them to harm the other person, and they didn't stop themselves.

It was some of the most "shocking" work on obedience we have ever seen. Milgram specifically reflected on the idea of "blind" obedience, especially the fact that people were willing to do some pretty rotten things simply because a person in a position of authority had told them to do so. The volunteers denied who they were and what they would ordinarily do—choosing right over wrong—all in the name of obedience.

Most of us when we hear about the study think we wouldn't have done what the people in the room did. We think we might have behaved differently. Don't be so sure. Two-thirds of Milgram's research subjects did it, and they were ordinary Yale students. And guess what? Maybe you don't shock strangers because of what someone tells you to do, but instead, you sort of "shock" yourself every day because of what others tell you. Over and over again, you deny what you want to do, who you want to be, how you want to live, what you know to be right, and even how you want to eat, all because of what others in your world—people who matter to you—want you to do. In general, most of us are blindly obedient to the wishes of others.

Just as an aside, Milgram's experiments could never be done today. It would not fall within the ethical guidelines we currently employ in research. Nonetheless, his research speaks volumes about what we do for others, even when we know something is not right (or perhaps even downright dangerous) for us, or for another person.

FOLLOWING THE TRIBE

The impact of stakeholders is actually captured in the classic work of Solomon Asch, a social psychologist, who examined conformity (which is a little different than the idea of obedience from Milgram—most of us may not think of ourselves as "obedient," but it's amazing how easily we conform). In his studies, Asch used a simple task in which a small group of subjects was shown a card with three lines of differing length on it. The subjects were then shown another white card that had one line on it, and they were to indicate which line on the card of three lines it was closest to in length. Turns out everyone in the "group" was told to give the wrong answer, except for the last person in the group, who was not "in" on the experiment. The right answer was GLARINGLY clear; nonetheless, in over a third of the cases, the poor test subject would go along with the others and give the same wrong answer they had provided. In general, the more people there were who gave the wrong answer, the more likely the last person would be to conform. Interestingly, even having just one person give the right answer would be enough to shift this tendency to conform, and the test subject would then be more likely to give the answer he or she knew to be right all along. Sometimes it just takes one stakeholder who encourages you to listen to yourself to keep you from blindly running with the tribe.

IDENTIFYING A STAKEHOLDER

Stakeholders are everywhere, and some are more powerful than others. Basically a stakeholder is *anyone whose opinion matters to you and influences your behavior and choices.* This means that stakeholders are family members, children, bosses, coworkers, neighbors, people in your religious community, and at a larger level, society as a whole.

If their opinion matters to you at all, in any way, then they are stakeholders. And if their input influences your behavior and your choices, they are really stakeholders. We are a social species, and as such, the opinions of others influence us; that is not going to change. But at the end of the day, there are stakeholders, and there are *stakeholders*. The critical issue becomes the degree to which you deny your spider senses and what you know is right for you in the name of your stakeholders.

Let's consider a few examples:

- You stay in a broken relationship or marriage because you don't want to lose your social network or hurt your children.

- You stay in a job that you hate and that feels bad because your spouse / partner expects you to earn a certain income, to maintain a certain quality of life.

- You get engaged and marry someone, even when you're not sure about it, to please your family and friends.

- You turn down a unique opportunity (travel, work, creative experience) that you have dreamed about because your family and close friends mock you for "wasting time" on something that doesn't pay, or doesn't pay enough.

- You eat an entire plate of food when you aren't hungry because you don't want to hurt your mother's feelings.

OUTGROWING A STAKEHOLDER

Stakeholder influences don't change over the course of a life as much as you would think. When you are a child, pleasing a parent drives your behavior. At some level that's a good thing; a good parent models healthy and appropriate behavior and teaches a child right from wrong. The child's inherent motivation to garner parental approval is how the child practices and learns pro-social and healthy behavior. But it gets delicate when the child is attempting to try out his wings and trust his gut. Again, the most basic example of this occurs at the table when the child is full and the parent says, "No, you're not."

As we get older, in some ways, those influences become more powerful, especially when we feel like we didn't get enough parental approval or presence early on. That connection, that attachment, is an essential part of human development. If we have a solid, secure, and healthy attachment to a caregiver during infancy and early childhood, it sets the tone for us to be better equipped to navigate the world and soothe ourselves. If we don't get it, we go looking for it—for the rest of our lives. We look for that approval and regard from our friends, teachers, lovers, spouses, coworkers, and bosses. And if you reflect on some of the most broken relationships of your life, you will notice that in most of them, you were (or are) blindly seeking approval and regard—in other words, sticking it out and behaving in ways to please them.

There is a poignant scene in Edith Wharton's novel *The Age of Innocence*—the ultimate stakeholder novel—that takes this on. The main character, Newland Archer, gives up the love of his life and an authentic life with the well-matched Countess Olenska for the simpler, but more appropriate (according to his stakeholders) Mae Welland. Newland's spider senses appear to be spot-on about the countess and his less-than-optimal match with Mae, but ultimately his tribe of stakeholders wins. He learns to silence his spider senses, and he and the countess forever part ways. Years later when Newland's children are grown, and Mae has died, his son says:

> "She said she knew we were safe with you, and always would be, because once, when she asked you to, you'd given up the thing you most wanted." Archer received this strange communication in silence. His eyes remained unseeingly fixed on the thronged sunlit square below the window. At length he said in a low voice: "She never asked me." (288)

This scene always affects me profoundly because it potently addresses the point that stakeholders don't always directly ask for what they want, but somehow we anticipate and deliver anyhow. Wharton eloquently refers to the work of the stakeholders as a "conspiracy," and for many of us who feel as though we stopped living our own lives a long time ago, it does feel like a conspiracy.

I have a hope that every human being comes to this realization—that when it's all over, your stakeholders may never thank you for your sacrifices—before it is too late. It's tragic, the number of times I have heard people come to this place much later in life, after they "stuck it out" for the kids, worked for the gold watch and retirement dinner, and realized that the stakeholders were either dead, gone, or didn't care, and that they had given up on dreams, hopes, and opportunities blindly. Don't let this happen to you. However, don't think it will be easy to walk away from these stakeholders and honor yourself, because you'll learn as you continue reading, there *will* be a body count.

STAKEHOLDERS AREN'T LABELED

Everyone who comes into your life is a potential stakeholder. Some stakeholders are what I term "heavy" stakeholders. For example, there are your parents and spouses or partners—the ones who really weigh you down and can scramble your signals in a powerful way. However, anyone can be a stakeholder, even someone who just briefly passes through your life. I have felt guilty in restaurants when a waitress looked disappointed when I didn't finish my meal (as though I was communicating that it wasn't good) and didn't want to take it home. I often have to convince a waitress that the food was indeed delicious, but simply too much. In that moment, a waitress is a stakeholder. This speaks to the power of any stakeholder. There was a time, and sometimes still is, that the person in me that lives to please even a perfect stranger such as a waitress would have eaten more or taken it home to do so. Think about that: I have, and I'm sure you have too, wanted to please someone I have never met and will likely never meet again.

Our hidden stakeholders are tricky because we like to envision ourselves as strong, independent-minded creatures. Most of us are pretty aware of how the heavy stakeholders influence us, but we must remain mindful of the hidden stakeholders—those whom we don't think have any power, but who are silently influencing us. Their hidden nature gives them even more power. Since we may not be mindful or aware of their influence, we may actually believe we are acting in accordance with what we want, when we are in fact behaving in ways to please those hidden folks. And we are artful at crafting complex rationalizations at such times.

ALWAYS TRYING TO PLEASE

We are hardwired to please. Human beings are a social and tribal species; indeed, our brains are wired in a way that almost requires us to share some of the cognitive burden with others.

At one time, tribes were great, and, in fact, necessary. We divided up the responsibilities. Some people collected the grain, some raised the kids, some hunted for meat, some were the healers; and while the tribe was efficient and essential, the survival of the tribe often depended on people denying their own individual needs and drives. Today, life's decisions are more complex than ever; we are not in simple survival mode, and we face endless choices—choices we are often better equipped to make if we aren't numbed by our stakeholders.

Stakeholders aren't all bad. They can be an important sounding board, they can bring us perspective on the basis of their experiences, and they can teach us. The problem is that it's tricky to let just that part in and not get lost in wanting to "do right" by them. Rare is the person that just gives of themselves to you, but then does not have an investment in an outcome. Rare is that person who can give you unconditional support and information, love you and respect you for you, but encourages you to make your own choices, even if they do not agree with you.

ARE YOU SURE?

There are few questions so insensitive, so arrogant, and so dangerous to spider senses.

"Are you sure?" can be used in a variety of ways. There are obviously the innocuous uses. Perhaps you go to a restaurant and your dining companion has eaten there but you have not. He has had the steak and told you that it's not good. In this case, "Are you sure?" could be a useful stopgap, although it would be followed by "The steak here is actually not very good."

Where "Are you sure?" gets to be problematic is when you are engaged in big-ticket decision-making, particularly the kind of decision-making that may have a body count, like starting or ending a relationship, job-related decisions, having children, expensive purchases. Sadly, we also do this to our kids, the very little people who are learning to trust their spider senses, and we scramble them all the time.

Short of the small group of people who are truly impulsive—spending their inheritance on a sports car, running off to Vegas despite being on unemployment—and who will not be affected by all the "Are you sure's?" in the world, this question is basically an indictment of your spider senses.

In general, for many people, when they are pondering a big decision such as a divorce, they have thought long and hard about it. It is like an iceberg; most of the decision was made under the water, privately, out of the sight of others, too painful and frightening to utter out loud. By the time most people get to the point of discussing it with others, they have done most of the heavy lifting and are taking their idea out for launch. They are scared, they feel isolated, and they are worried about what the world will think.

They are sure. And even if they aren't, another person's so-called questioning isn't going to change their mind; it's only going to fire up their anxiety.

Think about it for yourself: When you finally came to a decision about something big, how many times had you denied your spider senses, tried to talk yourself into and out of it, turned the decision around in your mind, anticipated what your stakeholders would want, let fear silence you, let childhood fairy tales and personal scripts thwart you? Then one day, if you were fortunate, you broke through all of that, used the data, let your spider senses guide you, and made a decision. Even though no one knew the rest of that process, you were sure about it. Yet, one "Are you sure?" could still bring you to your knees.

"Are you sure?" scrambles spider senses like few questions do. "Are you sure?" in essence says, "Do you really know what you want?" At the dinner table it asks the question, "Are you really full?"

The problem is that we often take these big-ticket choices to our stakeholders. And stakeholders are the choir that loves to sing encore after encore of "Are you sure?"

So what are we to do? This question is almost hardwired in us after years of being asked the question and years of asking it ourselves. The day I wrote these words, I myself was asked the question three times, had two patients struggle with people doing this to them, my partner was asked this question, and a friend was asked this question. That was just one day.

So how are we supposed to deal with "Are you sure?"—with what I call the "Medusa Trap"?

In Greek mythology, if you looked at the Gorgon Medusa—the rather frightening demoness, the snaky-haired woman—you turned to stone. Perseus managed to kill her and then he beheaded her. Athena placed her head on her shield and anyone who looked at her shield turned to stone. The techniques below can turn your "Are you sure?" askers to stone.

Basically, when they ask you "Are you sure?," they are asking the question of themselves. When they question whether you're sure you want to leave your relationship or marriage, they may be questioning the health of their own. When they ask if you're sure you are full, they may still be hungry, or have their own issues with food. When they ask if you're sure you want to leave your law career to become a musician, they likely have their own ambivalence about their life choices.

The next time you are "Are you sure-d?," turn their shield on them—turn them into stone. Realize that you are hearing their doubts. Continue to honor your own voice.

So what can you do when you hear "Are you sure?" First of all, take a moment, breathe, and realize you *are* sure. Then try one of these statements on for size. They acknowledge gratitude for another person's concern (which is what "Are you sure?" often is), they let you vent your fear, and they acknowledge the inherent challenges. They let you put down the gloves and refuse to turn this into a dialogue about someone else's script for you, but instead, let you own your process.

- "Thank you for asking."

- "It's never easy to make a big decision."

- "It's scary, but I am sure."

- "Yes."

- "I'm aware of the challenges, thanks for caring."

And you may be on both sides of this weapon. What if you are an "Are you sure?" asker? How do you stop yourself? What else can you ask instead? How about:

- "Tell me what's going on."

- "How are you feeling?"

- "That must be challenging."

- "How long has this been going on?"

- "How can I help?"

Imagine all the times you have heard "Are you sure?" What if you'd heard one of the abovementioned options in its place? Instead of defending yourself, or making your friend defend herself, you open up a dialogue. You stop projecting your hopes for yourself onto your friend and support her so she can get to where she needs to go. She will share her ambivalence with you organically. Few big decisions are made without some doubt. And at the end of the day, it is her life. Her spider senses are her own, just as yours are your own. You cannot steer someone else's ship, and if you think you can, it's an arrogant assumption.

In a particularly delightful scene from the movie *Beginners,* the elderly father is telling his son that he intends to move his new partner into his home after being widowed. The son asks his father, "Are you sure?," and the father responds with "Just be happy for me." That may be one of the best "Are you sure?" responses out there; it is simple, elegant, and truthful.

And if you think this is just an amateur error, let's take a look at how even people who know better can "Are you sure?" you.

I recently sat with someone who has been struggling with a challenging marriage. The marriage had lasted about sixteen years, and it was characterized by a manipulative, charming, and intimidating husband and a fearful wife whose self-esteem had eroded significantly after years of insults. They had faced some unique challenges in their marriage, and the wife had come to the realization several years earlier that it was over. But as most people do, she tried to empty her plate—she tried to do everything possible to save the marriage, including things that she was ethically and morally opposed to. Her life felt like a prison, and she reported a sense of dread and doom when she heard her husband's car in the driveway at the end of the day. She felt useless as a mother, and, increasingly, as a person. But they were masters at window dressing—the tableau of the Christmas card with the smiling kids and suntanned parents, Facebook posts, and pictures about their life together. Anyone looking at this mess from the outside would have envied these two people, their children, and the life they had constructed.

She spent years in therapy with her husband, trying to work on it. That's good; therapy is good, right?

Be aware of whom your stakeholders are. Even your hired guns can let you down. Sadly for this woman, even though their therapist had been privy to many of the tribulations in their marriage, he had his own agenda, and was very pro-marriage, or perhaps pro-man or anti-change—who the hell knows? He was a big fan of taking people who were already full and sending them back to the buffet table. After years of anguish and some final episodes of humiliation, after years of trying to finish everything on her plate, she asked for a divorce. Her husband called her every name in the book and issued all kinds of cruel threats around custody and finances. The woman bravely went into a therapy session that her husband elected not to attend and told their therapist what she had done.

His first question to her was "Are you sure?"

She was devastated. She thought the one person who had heard every terrible thing, things she did not want to share with the world in general, would at least want to hear her out. He was the one person who was supposed to support her process of decision-making. Even people who should know better (her therapist) can't turn off this narcissistic switch. (In my practice, I work from a humanistic, existential model of acceptance and unconditional respect—I believe those are the conditions of growth, make for good parenting, make for good relationship-ing, friendship-ing, you name it. "Are you sure?" doesn't belong in a therapy room—or any other room, for that matter.)

The nice thing was that after she'd gained the courage it took to finally stand strong and walk away from her marriage, she was also able to stand strong against the therapist, looking him squarely in the eye and saying, "Yes, I'm sure."

Instead of "Are you sure-ing?" each other, it's time we started "assuring" each other and ourselves. Put that question away forever, and the next time you hear it, smile wisely and stand strong.

WHY DO THEY HAVE A STRANGLEHOLD ON US?

Pleasing stakeholders starts early—and lasts a lifetime. It feels good to make someone else happy; it is why we purchase gifts, send cards, and share good words. Not only does it infuse someone else's life with joy, but when we do something good for someone else, we're also filled with good feelings, and that's powerful. Pleasing other people is easier, and it's a way to avoid conflict. When you look at the short list of the main things in life that people want to avoid, it would include fear, strong emotion, and conflict. Think of the number of times you have swallowed strong feelings, disappointment, hopes, aspirations, and just plain good ideas in the name of avoiding conflict. We cave in to our stakeholders in an effort to keep our path smooth.

Sometimes you keep going back to toxic stakeholders out of guilt, self-sabotage, an excuse to quit, or simply out of familiarity. This means that the weight you can't drop, the relationship you don't want, the relationship you do want, the job you don't like—it's not your problem, and you can pawn it off on someone else. However, in many cases, your stakeholders may not change. They may still "Are you sure?" you, and question you, or kill your dreams, or shut you down. Then the ball is in your court. If you keep going back in, it's futile, and the equivalent of hitting yourself over the head with a hammer—there is no point, unless your goal is to hurt yourself.

I want to point out that not all stakeholders are bad. You might have good stakeholders, ones whose advice you really value. You might want to consult with the uncle who is a doctor, or the cousin who's in the field in which you want to work. It's good to check in with them and get their viewpoints, but then you need to check back in with yourself. Don't outsource the responsibility for your decision by blaming them if something goes wrong. Own your choices. Consult for certain, and weigh their words, but trust you and make sure you are the ultimate decider of your life. Stakeholders are a two-way street when it comes to taking responsibility; you need to take responsibility for relying on them at appropriate times, but regardless of whether or not you turn to them, ultimately you need to take responsibility for your own decisions. This will become easier to do as you learn to rely on your spider senses.

Many of the most painful and difficult decisions in my life involved a fork in the road. Each time, my spider senses were 100 percent dead-on, pointing me in a certain direction. Unfortunately, that turn in the road would often require me to hurt, disappoint, or otherwise enter into conflict with a stakeholder. I would anguish over the decision, mostly because I wanted to avoid the negative experience I would have to manage with my stakeholders, even though the right decision was as clear as day. The potency of wanting to avoid a conflict or disappointment with a stakeholder often led me to make some big mistakes. Many times I did the "wrong" thing, caving in to the stakeholder and walking away from opportunities, dreams, and healthy options. Initially, in the minutes, hours, and days after making the decision, my first emotion was relief. But, that is paradoxical. How could violating a spider sense result in relief? Shouldn't it do the opposite? In these cases where I had to choose between pleasing a stakeholder(s) versus honoring myself, the initial praise, love, adoration, and congratulations I would get for "doing the right thing" was intoxicating. Or the relief I would experience from getting them off my back allowed me to return to the familiar comfort of the usual, the reinforcement of praise, to avoid change. But then about three to five days later, this relief would be replaced by dread, and the words "What have I done?" would begin thrumming through my soul.

Stakeholders are almost as powerful as drugs if you think about it. People use drugs because in the short term, they make them feel good—they can numb, excite, create pleasure—but in the long term, the crash is dreadful. Many substance abusers report that drug use trumps their spider senses. In most cases, they knew drugs were messing up their lives, but it was just easier to keep doing them and ultimately, their brains craved and almost "needed" them. We crave our stakeholders, and just like drugs, they can definitely scramble our spider senses. So in that way, stakeholders are an addiction of sorts, and that is why they are a hard habit to break.

At the end of the day, if we have to take sole responsibility for a decision (including what we put into our mouths)—if we can't pin it on stakeholders—then we have to go down with the ship if it sinks. That's a tough one. It is certainly a luxury to listen to our stakeholders and when things go south, be able to say, "Hey, you guys told me to do it this way—it's not my fault." Outsourcing blame is one of the ways our stakeholders get in and are allowed to place a stranglehold on us. If they can share the blame, then that makes them very useful. It's not necessarily functional, but it gives us a glimpse into one of the big reasons stakeholders can be so powerful.

IDENTIFYING STAKEHOLDERS

Identifying a stakeholder requires being honest with yourself. Over time, as you begin to see how many people are telling you how to live, you will wonder when you stopped being you. Not all stakeholders are the same: some can silence your spider senses, and others can remind you to listen to them. When you identify stakeholders in your life, think about the following:

- How do you feel about their opinions?
- Do you feel responsible for them?
- How would you feel about defying their opinions?
- How would your life be different without them?
- How often do you turn to them for guidance?
- How do they influence your behavior?

Your spider senses have a lot to do with identifying your stakeholders. In an ideal world, we would listen to ourselves before we'd let other people in. How many times have you met someone only to have those hairs on the back of your neck stand up and make you feel uncomfortable? Our culture of "Don't judge" and "Get along with everyone" can often lead us to silence those early reactions. People often become stakeholders because we let them in too deep, against our better judgment. Now, some people are along for the ride right from the beginning, like family and childhood friends, but after a point, you are your own gatekeeper (which we'll address more closely in chapter 5).

The table below breaks down the different kinds of stakeholders and allows you to reflect on their power and influence. Think about where your stakeholders fit into this matrix.

DIFFERENT TYPES OF STAKEHOLDERS

TYPE OF STAKEHOLDER	EXAMPLES	CHARACTERISTICS
Heavy stakeholders	Parents, spouses / intimate partners, children, and, in some cases, siblings.	Have a longstanding hold on you; their opinions are significant and influential and your behavior has significant implications for them.
Daily stakeholders	Friends, family, close coworkers.	These can also be heavy stakeholders, and are knitted into the daily fabric of your life; while they may not always have the same powerful hold over you, their regular presence does influence your choices, and their opinions can influence your behaviors.
Circumstantial stakeholders	People you are forced to interact with through circumstance—neighbors, coworkers, members of clubs and religious communities, fellow parents at a school, fellow students.	These are people you may have very regular contact with, but whom you may not choose to have in your life otherwise. However, because they are part of the landscape of your life—perhaps only temporarily—they do influence behaviors and choices, especially in the settings where you interact with them.

DIFFERENT TYPES OF STAKEHOLDERS *CONTINUED*

TYPE OF STAKEHOLDER	EXAMPLES	CHARACTERISTICS
Stranger stakeholders	People you may just interact with for a brief period, and may never see again (or rarely); this can include service professionals (clerks, cashiers, waitresses), people you meet in passing.	A person who is only in your life for a short period may not seem like a stakeholder, but they may weigh in on a food choice, a purchase, or your behavior. It's important to identify your vulnerability to these stakeholders, because it may lead you to silence your spider senses even at times when familiar stakeholders aren't around.
Toxic stakeholders	These can be any of the above; they leave you unsettled, and you often walk away from interactions feeling dejected and pessimistic.	These are people who kill your dreams, infect you with their fears, insult you, and "Are you sure?" you. These folks tend to be major time-suckers; they bring drama, negative emotions, and easily misinterpret other people's words as rejection or criticism. A mistake such as not calling them back can lead to weeks of recriminations and accusations, and much time is spent dealing with and soothing them and spending obligatory time with them—time you will never get back and rarely grow from.

DIFFERENT TYPES OF STAKEHOLDERS *CONTINUED*		
TYPE OF STAKEHOLDER	**EXAMPLES**	**CHARACTERISTICS**
Unconditional stakeholders	Can be any of the above, but they are people who stand by you, offer advice when asked, and listen.	These are the rarest of the stakeholders, and they are the keepers— the ones who listen and who are able to offer advice without looping themselves into the equation. They are there for you unconditionally, even if they do not always agree with or understand your choice. They allow you to respond to and cultivate your spider senses. Ironically, these people are often so easy and loving that they don't suck our time and as such we don't get the benefits of these interactions as often as we should (in marked contrast to the toxic stakeholders).

HOW TO CONSUME YOUR STAKEHOLDERS

Every stakeholder represents a choice. You can choose:

- whether you listen to them,
- whether you ask for their advice,
- whether you let them in, or
- whether you walk away from them.

To borrow a food analogy: We have to learn how to "consume" our stakeholders. Sometimes we may crave certain calorie-rich or "unhealthy" foods, but we can learn to eat them in smaller portions or in a healthier context (e.g., cutting a burger in half, eating it without the bun, or not getting cheese on it). Sometimes we want to be with our stakeholders, but they may not be optimal to share a dream with or ask advice of, so you need to become skilled at learning how to turn to them, enjoy them, and be with them without letting them thwart your decision-making process.

Over time, you will find that you have organically pulled away from the toxic stakeholders, and hopefully learned new ways of interacting with the others. If you start honoring your spider senses, some of your stakeholders may walk away from you. This happened to me. When I made some big-ticket decisions in my life around ending my marriage, the body count was high. My family didn't think I should be chasing my dreams because I had children. They viewed my divorce as a family failure.

Now, a few years later, some of them have circled back, and certainly I consume them more cautiously. But by honoring myself, I am able to enter back into relationships with them from a more-informed space, and consume them in a different way. It hurt when people walked away from me for honoring my spider senses. And then, as it often happens, one day it stopped hurting. The new life that bloomed, with the toxic players out, remains a daily miracle to me. It still hurts sometimes to have shifted relationships with parents and to have lost friends, but to have gained a life and the strength that comes from that, to be able to say no to seconds, to mean-spirited words, to toxic people—that in and of itself becomes self-sustaining.

THE COMMON THREAD

Stakeholders are simply people and organizations that matter to us. There are many reasons they matter, and these include the following:

- They are familiar—they look like us, sound like us, or have a similar background to us.
- They remind us of the past.
- They are powerful.
- They care about us.
- They love us.
- They spend time with us.
- They share our interests.

Most stakeholders have at least one of these qualities, and most have three or more. They can't get in close unless there is a hook. We often don't engage with people who are too different from us, because we gravitate to that which is familiar. We mate with people who are like us; our tribes are comprised of people who share characteristics with us. People who like sports hang out with sports fans, people who love food hang out with other foodies, and people who support our assumptions about ourselves (good or bad) are the ones we keep close.

One way to keep your stakeholders' assumptions about you in check is to change the assumptions you make about yourself. Fix that and your stakeholders will change with you (or they will leave).

STAKEHOLDERS ARE JUST PEOPLE

The concept of stakeholders resonates strongly with my patients. As they tell me about the people who populate their social network, I ask questions that illuminate for me how those stakeholders may have led to where my patients now find themselves, or how they contribute to their ongoing difficulties with decision-making. I am simply helping the patient with a game of connect the dots.

Initially, pulling the mask off of stakeholders is often met with a defensive reaction from people I work with; they will defend their stakeholders, and that makes sense. Their defensive reactions often speak volumes about the power of their stakeholders, and the fears that surround angering them, losing them, or taking responsibility for decisions. I have had patients stay in marriages out of pity, stay in contact with abusive parents out of guilt, not fire incompetent employees out of loyalty, and give up opportunities because their families labeled them as selfish. We start by identifying the connections, and I make it clear to them that if it is so easy to lose their stakeholder by choosing something that will lead them to growth, then perhaps that relationship was too weak to maintain.

But remember that all stakeholders do not hold you back, and those unconditional stakeholders can be game changers and make you brave enough to make changes, whether at the dinner table or in other areas of your lives. If you can start listening to yourself, you too will become an unconditional stakeholder for others. And the freedom you will experience from honoring your spider senses will benefit others, or as more eloquently stated by the poet Charles Bukowski, "the free soul is rare, but you know it when you see it—basically because you feel good, very good, when you are near or with them."

ADVICE ON ADVICE

The fact is, it's damned near impossible to give advice to someone without it being what we want for ourselves. Thus, when you ask for advice, remember that most likely the other person is telling you what they would do for themselves, not necessarily what is best for you. This can make for some tricky business, because we can often talk ourselves out of what we know is truly right for us. Here's an example: I have a friend who was really working hard at losing weight. She had curbed her calories, especially when it came to alcohol. She worked in an office that often gathered for drinks after work. She joined her regular gang and when her friend asked her if she wanted a second martini, she said no, she'd have club soda. That's good decision-making; it was hard, but she did it anyway. She decided club soda was a better choice because a second martini meant more calories, and probably mindless eating to follow. Her friend wasn't cutting calories (although she should have been), but as a stakeholder, she wanted a partner in crime. The not-on-a-diet-right-now friend crossed her arms and said sulkily, "Fine, I won't have another one either," but with that, my friend caved in to her guilt and joined her for another cocktail.

Do we ever get to a place when we are "stakeholder-free"? I don't think so. We are a social species, and feedback is often an essential part of decision-making. Our stakeholders are an important part of our lives. Perhaps it seems like calling them stakeholders dehumanizes them, because at the end of the day they love us, they support us, cry with us, laugh with us, fill us with happiness, anger, and a million other emotions. The key becomes honoring your spider senses while allowing these relationships to unfold and exist. Because with time, the beautiful thing that happens is that when you honor yourself, fight the good fight, take the chances, integrate the advice, but ultimately trust yourself, you model something very important for your stakeholders. Once they see you succeed and excel and shine, some of them will start taking those chances themselves.

I think I have inspired more people to successful weight loss not through my words, but through my life—through not only a successful loss of eighty-five pounds, but by watching me take chances, make changes, honor my voice, face down my fears, and pursue my dream. In the short term your stakeholders may recoil at your willingness to be you, and some may leave, but those who stay will have seen the authentic you, and will learn through observation how to listen to their own beautiful voices.

THE WHY

Taking on stakeholders is tough, which is why I remind patients of the wide range of responses available to them, from walking away to learning how to work around them while honoring their spider senses. Many times I have looked at a scenario from the outside and reflected on the fact that if we could just get distance between the patient and a specific family member (or just eliminate the relationship altogether), we would make quantum leaps. But evaporating human relationships is not that simple, and so the task becomes one of figuring out how to help clients find ways to integrate stakeholders into their lives in a way that facilitates growth and allows their spider senses to blossom.

Part of taking them on is identifying them and their role in your life. It helps you to organize yourself, and lets you be on alert when you interact with certain kinds of stakeholders. If you can be mindful when you encounter your different kinds of stakeholders, you will be better prepared to keep your spider senses on point. Some stakeholders are people we have known all our lives, and some are strangers. They are also the messages we receive from the world, advertisers, and television. Living to please is like living a half-life. In my years of working with clients with disordered eating and weight problems, and from my own story of weight loss, I've learned that one thing is clear: People who struggle with weight also struggle with the desire to please others.

Food is often consumed in an interpersonal context. Our first lessons around food often involved eating to please. In many cultures, hospitality is expressed via overeating or piling on more food. Restaurants give oversized portions, and even though we don't know the chef or waitress, we eat to please them, or our dining companions. Pleasing others is hard work—and we often do it so we can feel in control of our environments. It gives us a way to organize our behavior, and it also teaches us to quiet our own instincts and respond to another's cues. Females in much of the world are socialized to please—to please their elders, play cooperatively, obey their husband—and while feminism has made a dent in this, women and pleasing are still like two peas in a pod, and weight-related dyscontrol is still very much the province of women.

If we eat to please, cook to please, and then, in the midst of this pleasing parade, feel so out of control that we also eat to soothe, numb, cheer up, shut down, and distract, food becomes a multipurpose drug. An easy way to break that cycle is to stop eating for anyone but yourself. The food you eat nourishes you, fills you, and only you know what you want or when you have had enough. Just as no one else can tell you if you are hot or cold or tired or angry or happy, no one can tell you how and when to eat.

THE NOW

Grab your journal and a pen. This exercise is something you do over time, and I'm aware this list will keep growing.

STEP 1:

Write down the names of the people who influence your daily life: people from your past; people who have influenced your decision-making during the last year; the people you turn to with good news and bad, or big-ticket decisions.

Don't hesitate to go to your cell-phone contacts, Facebook page, and address book and pull names from there. What will be interesting is the order of the names. Make note of whether a pattern emerges (for example: Do more toxic stakeholders jump out at you initially? Do you list family members initially? Do you wait until later in your list to write down coworkers?).

STEP 2:

Beside each name, I want you to write down your relationship to each person in the list, and then define the type of stakeholder they represent to you (people can be more than one—for example, Mom may be both Heavy and Toxic):

- Heavy
- Daily
- Circumstantial
- Stranger
- Toxic
- Unconditional

STEP 3:

List the actual decisions they have each influenced you to make (e.g., where you went to college, the car you purchased, who you married, where you live).

STEP 4:

Relationship rating: This is completely subjective, but using a scale of 1 to 10, where 10 is indicative of a relationship that you deeply value and is characterized by support, and 1 is a relationship that is abusive (in any way), toxic, and undermining, rate each relationship. You are your own reference here, but it will be important to note whether higher ratings are associated with people who allow your spider senses to flourish. Since this exercise is a work in progress, I want you to use it as a way to monitor change in how stakeholders affect your spider senses.

Stakeholder Dictionary

When you make a big decision, whatever it is, make one of these lists for the people you spoke to about that decision. By doing this you create a personal "stakeholder dictionary." Stakeholder influences are so woven into the daily fabric of our lives that we often don't recognize where we end and they begin. Step one to fixing this is breaking down how they influence you and your spider senses.

CHECK-IN: STAKEHOLDERS

Once or twice a week (or daily, if you wish), reflect on how a stakeholder impacted your decision-making. Indicate whether they pushed you with or against your spider senses.

Practice "Are you sure" responses. I can all but guarantee that you will be "Are you sure-d" a few times per week. Try out one of the responses and see how it is received. Also, when you feel tempted to "Are you sure?" someone else, try out one of the new responses instead.

CHAPTER 3

The Not-So-Golden Rules

The golden rule is that there are no golden rules.
—George Bernard Shaw

What if we were to create a modern-day mélange fairy tale for a girl in our society?

> Once upon a time there was a gorgeous little girl. She was born into a loving family with a biological mother and father that loved each other very much. They lived in a big and beautiful home, and she was a wonderful student and a gifted musician and athlete. She had siblings and all were happy and healthy. They ate all of the food on their plates and never complained.
>
> The girl attended an excellent university where she met and dated lots of eligible young men. She dated a particularly nice one during her last year. He was from a family just like hers, and went on to develop his career as she explored her career interests as well. Over time they moved in together and decided to get married. He bought her a wonderful big ring, and they had a wonderful big wedding. He was a success and she wanted babies, so she decided to stay at home in their beautiful home with their beautiful babies.
>
> And of course, they lived happily ever after.

Short of a glass slipper or a poisoned apple, isn't this how we think all stories should progress? And shouldn't they all end exactly like this?

Now, let's really delve into Aesop and Hans Christian Andersen and the Brothers Grimm and Disney, and the fables our parents and grandparents and communities told us. Let's recall the epics and the fireside stories, the fairy tales of our youth that filled our heads with images of how things should be. Add the basic rules of order driven by commandments, mythology, and religion—tales that were often told to us at bedtime that we took into our dream worlds and that set the tone for our fears, wishes, and lives.

I must say that one of the most powerful stories for me was "The Red Shoes." In this story by Hans Christian Andersen, a little girl from a poor family gets one new pair of shoes each winter. Because they can afford just one pair, she always gets the same brown leather ones. One year she and her family walk in front of the store and she sees a divine pair of red shoes, beautiful, but simply unsuitable for the cold months and work ahead. Oh, but the young girl covets the red shoes, and since she loves to dance, she imagines how they would allow her to realize her dreams of dancing. She is a good girl, and so on this year her parents entrust her to go to the store with the hard-won money and purchase her shoes herself.

She gets to the store and the power of the red shoes is too much. She figures shoes are shoes, so she gets them. She wears them out of the store and finds that in these shoes she can dance more amazingly than she has ever danced before. She dances through the fields and meadows, all the way home. But as she nears home she finds that she can't stop. She keeps dancing right past her home and back to the store, but she still can't stop. As darkness falls she gets closer to home and is nearly falling down with exhaustion. Her father, a woodcutter, looks down at her feet and sees what has happened. There was no way to take off the shoes, so he cuts off her feet and they go dancing off into the woods. The punishment for her hubris? A life without feet.

I was terrified upon hearing that story as a child, but listen I did, right into adulthood. I was scared to death of breaking the rules, taking a chance, defying my elders, because then I might literally lose my limbs, or worse. Think of the lessons and teachings we learned from very early on:

- Never defy your elders.
- Remain quiet.

- Wait for fate to cast a hand.

- Honor duty.

All of these lessons, like "Eat everything on your plate," are focused on order and control.

I was raised on the even more heavy-handed tale of duty dictated by Rama and Sita in the Ramayana. Rama is forced into exile for a very long time. Nobody believes Sita will remain his devoted wife while he is gone, in part because nobody knew if he was even still alive. But Sita was devoted because Rama was her guy, so she lived her life in devotion to him throughout his exile. When he finally returned, he was named King of Ayodhya and Sita, his queen.

It was known to the kingdom that temptations had been sent her way to test her throughout his exile, all of which Sita had withstood. When Rama went to take his throne it was very important to the citizenry that their queen be pure—so they asked her to succumb to a test. Rama should have been a stand-up guy and told them that he knew she had been devoted, but as many do, he caved in to his stakeholders and sheepishly asked her to take the test. He told her that if she were devoted then she would pass anyhow, and it would all be okay. She, of course, dutifully bowed her head and said, "Of course, my lord."

The test required her to walk through fire. If she was pure, the fire would not burn her, and if she was sullied, well, then she would burn to death. She walked through the fire and she lived, emerging unscathed.

Rama breathed a sigh of relief, knowing she was devoted, and was ready to face the people with their new queen. Here's the problem (and they never told me this feminist postscript when I was young): After she passed the test, she left and returned to Mother Earth. She figured that he should have known her to be pure and he should never have caved to the pressure of the stakeholders to make her prove her devotion. Sita was, in some ways, the original authentic feminist. But at the end of the day, this parable is about blind devotion and duty to stakeholders.

The rules of duty and devotion still pervade much of what I do, and it's likely that commandments, fables, and myths about "happily ever after" still drive much of what you do. These childhood teachings were the first way we organized our lives. Writers, especially Bruno Bettelheim, talk about how fairy tales both frighten us and provide structure for our world.

Childhood stories stick with us because they taught us how to organize our worlds, what to want, and what to think. Happily-ever-after leads many a little girl to dream of a fairy-tale wedding. In addition, our childhood myths gave us insight into how to please our stakeholders, and if children want to do one thing, they want to please, and they want positive regard. Those stories contained implicit messages about how to please the world. And while we are able to intellectually argue away the simplicity of these lessons, where the rubber meets the road, they still guide our thinking.

Breaking childhood teachings is never easy, and in essence, they are like white noise that can sometimes stop us from listening to ourselves, or having to listen to ourselves. (Remember: It is easier to maintain the status quo than to make a change; even if the status quo is awful, many people still choose to stay in it.) If we are able to take the risk of acting in defiance of a golden rule or fairy tale while acting in accordance with our spider senses, and then have a successful experience, that becomes an enormous brick in the wall of learning to honor our spider senses.

Imagine being raised with the "Winners never quit" line and the idea that success is measured monetarily. Then you decide to quit a financially plush but soul-numbing job at a prestigious firm because your heart, mind, soul, and spider senses are saying, "Run away!" Despite every childhood teaching telling you otherwise, you do so. You pursue your dream that honors you but may not bring the money or prestige. You struggle, and then the dream is realized. Perhaps you don't get rich, but each day you awaken emboldened by the possibility. Each decision that follows from this one is less and less likely to be influenced by the golden rules.

The first few breaks from the golden rules are hard, because they feel like flying without a net. Then, once you get your wings and trust your spider senses, the freedom will feel like flying. One criticism I hear is, "Won't people just walk away from everything if they do this, if they stop listening to these golden rules?" On the contrary; because they will be better decision-makers or gatekeepers, they will be more likely to make good choices on the way in and be less likely to feel compelled to walk away or be conflicted and unhappy about the choices later on.

REWRITING YOUR FAIRY TALE

As information streams into our world in new ways, the new progenitor of fairy tales in our world is the media, particularly reality television and the mountain of Internet imagery. In some ways, at least in the food world, the lessons are trickier. Anorexic model on one billboard, thousand-calorie burger on the other. Cupcake competition on one channel, plastic surgery transformations on another. Photoshopped images of impossible beauty next to supersized meals. The juxtaposition of food imagery is even more confusing than simple rules about clean plates, happily ever after, and not rocking the boat.

What if the stories were re-rendered? What if the fairy tale read as follows:

> Once upon a time a wee girl who grew up in the shadow of the palace found herself in a difficult life, caring for cruel stepsisters and a stepmother, and befriending the various rodents that populated her quarters. On the night of the big ball, a fairy godmother intervened and turned the dirty-faced girl into a dazzling specimen of womanhood. The young girl enchanted the prince, who fell in love with her, and when she dashed away at midnight, he vowed to use the shoe she left behind to find her.
>
> He did find her, and they married. She moved into the palace and, while he was doing his princely duties, she launched an initiative to ensure that no little girl would ever find herself in such a situation as hers. But her work increasingly pulled her away from the prince, and once they had children, they grew apart. Apparently one night of dancing and a shoe hunt was not enough on which to build this relationship, and the princess realized that she was feeling curtailed by the bounds of her life. She and the prince went to counseling, but he was really looking for a different life than she was, and so to honor herself, she suggested that they consider a break.

My daughter recently asked, "Why doesn't Cinderella have a sequel?" It was a good question; fairy tales often stop with the happily ever after, leaving us to muse on what "ever after" looks like. Even when modernist revisions attempt sequels, they still typically end up in a happy committed place. And the tales rarely teach the harder lesson of when to cut bait. Famous investor Warren Buffett once said, "Should you find yourself in a chronically leaking boat, energy devoted to changing vessels is likely to be more productive than energy devoted to patching leaks." Rarely do the childhood lessons offer this as an option. The ones that stick are typically the ones that tell us to stick.

Why are childhood lessons so sticky? If someone told me today, "Winners never quit," would it have such an impact?

The lessons of childhood often stick with us because we took them on to please others, just like we would eat to please others. In fact, doing things to please others may be the most classical fairy tale we sell children. It makes sense; it makes the adults' lives and society's control easier if they can socialize children that way, and the fact is, *we* were socialized that way, so we continue doing it, generation after generation.

At the end of the day, the golden rules allow us to outsource responsibility. If we don't let our spider senses drive the train, then we also don't have to take responsibility.

So the lessons of childhood are:

- Finish everything on your plate.
- Winners never quit.
- Don't question your elders.
- The night is full of scary, unknown creatures.
- Avoid risk.
- Save for a rainy day.

These lessons are powerful because we did these things to please parents, teachers, communities, and society.

TAKE ON THE RULES

We grew up learning and listening to these myths, fairy tales, and rules. It's time to start breaking them and stop letting them blindly guide the choices you make and the life you live and the food you eat. Let's take a look at them, one by one, and come up with a new—and better—set of rules.

Quitters Never Win, Winners Never Quit

Remember this one? Now look at the biographies of some of the most successful men and women in politics, science, technology, and media who sometimes quit, walked away, and stopped throwing bad money after good. Steve Jobs, Oprah Winfrey, Johnny Carson, Henry Ford, Bill Gates, Joe Kennedy, and Steven Spielberg, to name a few. Sometimes they failed, and people told them they were unfit for the work they wanted to do. Some quit school, some left successful TV shows, and nearly all of them said that they trusted their guts and pursued what felt right. Research by Timothy Judge, a professor at Notre Dame, has revealed that success may actually be a product of being able to choose the path to quit while moving forward on another path with conviction. We can get so buried in other projects and tasks that we forget to pay attention to the right path for us. So even though the old saying says that quitters never win, research actually suggests otherwise. It's about knowing when and what to quit so that you can pay attention to the better path for you.

Perhaps the list we aren't as familiar with is comprised of the people who trusted their guts and may not have achieved success; in fact, they may have lost everything. But then, would the taste of regret be worse than not trying at all? While they may not be famous, I have spoken with several people who did take risks and quit a more-conventional lifestyle to honor their spider senses, but did not achieve success. Not one of them termed the experience a failure, with most of them acknowledging that they felt good and brave about trying, and that they often reflected on the many lessons they'd learned. *Quitter* is such an ugly word because it implies lack of effort, laziness, and lack of determination. Sometimes a quitter is someone who listens to an inner voice and makes a choice. And sometimes they win, and win big.

New rule: Sometimes you have to quit to win.

Don't Talk to Strangers

This is about the fear of what happens when we talk to the scary person who is different from us. Now, this lesson has some utility for kids, who are suggestible. There are predatory people out there, and that childhood archetype of the villain hanging about with a bag of candy is an oldie but a goodie. In teaching children prudence, we often make them reticent, as kids and adults, to boldly share their thoughts and views with others. We, as humans, are already wired to gravitate toward people who are similar to us, and that can be limiting. Or we wait until we are in safe settings—meeting people at work, or at parties where everyone is somehow connected through school, or the host.

Talking to strangers—people who are unlike us, who just come out of nowhere—can harness things within us, and lead us to opportunities that would not otherwise happen. Your spider senses often steer you right. If a stranger doesn't feel right, then don't approach, but sometimes that stranger who feels approachable could be worth the hello. Talking to strangers led me to my great love, to some fascinating travel opportunities, and some of my best life lessons.

New rule: Say hello to one stranger a day. At a minimum you will brighten someone's day, and there is the possibility that you may change a life. Maybe your own.

FAIRY-TALE EXPECTATIONS

If we just blindly subscribe to fables and fairy tales, we will find ourselves making decisions that may reflect what Aesop, Walt Disney, and the Brothers Grimm want for us, but not what we know is best for us. Many times the golden rules and myths can set unrealistic or unhealthy expectations for a situation. Happily ever after. Don't fly too close to the sun. Patience is always a virtue. Duty always carries clear rewards. Clean your plate.

Good Things Come to Those Who Wait

Typically this golden rule results in lost opportunity and lost time. Patience. That great childhood lesson: Patience is supposed to be a virtue. The American writer and satirist Ambrose Bierce calls patience "[a] minor form of despair, disguised as a virtue." Yet, most spiritual teachers and pundits—the Dalai Lama, Lao Tzu, Rilke, Mother Teresa—love patience. Is some of this quality necessary in life? Yes; you can't always run to the head of the line. But this teaching—that good things come to those who wait—often begets inaction and a drive to shelve hopes, dreams, and aspirations in the name of patience. Most of us know when it is time to just do it, and stop waiting, but the big spider-sense scramblers of stakeholders and fear often paralyze us. And then one day we look back on years lost, with lots of accumulated waiting. Society loves patience because it quiets the dissatisfaction of the masses. By turning waiting into a good thing, it makes it easier for the existing structures to either take their own sweet time to create necessary change, or to not change at all.

Too often, we convince ourselves to wait and put our heads down and work hard instead of trusting our guts and not waiting, but going for it. Never wait on a dream.

New rule: Stop waiting and do it. Today.

FAIRY TALES RULE OUR WORLD

Boy meets girl.

Picket fences.

Happily ever after.

Everyone gets married.

Notions like these can lead to poor decision-making and impact our gatekeeping, because we think we need to strive for certain fairy-tale rules.

Get Along with Everyone

Have you ever met someone and instantly the hairs on the back of your neck stand up? That's your spider senses kicking in and screaming at you. But instead of backing away quietly, what do you do? You listen to the replay of the voice of your kindergarten teacher, telling you that it's nice to give everybody a chance. That person, more often than not, will disappoint you, time and time again. And even though you keep trying not to be judgmental, you need to remember that it is more than okay not to like everyone. Life is short, and spending time with people you don't like is not a good use of time. We have to do it enough at work and with our families.

It might seem okay to tolerate everyone and to keep trying to get along with people, but by forcing yourself to sustain those relationships, you are bruising your spider senses in order to fulfill some summer-camp fantasy that everyone needs to get along. This also plays into the rescue fantasy. Many times people will ignore spider senses and let someone in whom they feel can be helped or rescued. I'm a psychologist and I work with lots of people; I can say with certitude that no one can be "rescued." A human being is not an engine that you rebuild. When you feel the freedom to walk away from people, and situations, you'll also feel more empowered to walk away from plates.

New rule: Don't throw bad money after good in any relationship— give it a chance, but if it stops fitting, or you stop growing in it, it's okay to let it go.

Be Seen, Not Heard

Ah yes, the denial of a soul. The classic life lesson that tells you to silence yourself because you recall that the most virtuous child was the one who did not speak. I remember a trip to India when I was a child. Trips to India were often characterized by long, meandering visits to relatives with few distractions. There were no video games or iPad movies for me to watch then. I remember being told how wonderful I was for sitting silently for two hours in someone's house. It was awful, and the longer I did it, the longer I went unnoticed. By the time we went to the next place, the silence wasn't cutting it, and I let loose and began misbehaving. I went against my spider senses earlier in the day by just sitting silent, and then went against them later in the day by misbehaving. The better lesson for me would have been to be seen and heard throughout the day so I could have better taken in the experiences around me.

Consider this: In essence, my behavior in the evening was like an eating binge after a day of not eating. Obviously, listening is good, but silencing your voice so as not to rock the boat, upset stakeholders, or communicate clearly is not acceptable. By trusting your gut, you will often communicate your thoughts, hopes, and wants instead of silencing your-self and your spider senses. People can only be seen if they are heard, so speak out appropriately, clearly, and strongly.

New rule: Sing loud and strong and be heard and seen. Trust your voice.

Save Your Pennies for a Rainy Day

I have seen people destroy themselves in the name of this principle. Most financial advisers will tell you that you cannot save enough, and that this process of saving has to start young. The mandate here is often to postpone a lot of life in the name of saving, so that someday when you are quite old and no longer working, you will have enough money to live. Now obviously there is some prudence to this. We live in a country where it is expensive and perhaps even downright dangerous to not have a health-care or financial safety net when you are older, because social security benefits are often not sufficient, and retirement benefits often do not provide enough during a time of life when health-care costs increase and employment opportunities may be limited.

That said, when exactly is one supposed to live? Again, what if you trust your gut? In general, most people who are free of problems that can impair financial decision-making, such as addictions, impulse-control disorders, or other mental illnesses, are able to see the bigger picture and not just capriciously spend money. I will note that shopping is the new eating, and many people spend and shop for the same reasons that other people eat. However, the perceived virtue of saving instead of spending can often lead people to take on much harder lives.

I have a friend who had a full-time job, as did her husband, and they had a large brood of children. This woman spent many years training in her specialized field, and she wanted to find a balance between working and having children. Her spider senses told her that if she took ten years off to raise her children, she would not be able to stay in the profession she valued. So despite the prohibitive cost, she and her husband retained a full-time child-care person at home. I foolishly did not, and it really took a toll not only on me and my husband at the time, but on our children as well. She had no more money than I did; in fact, she may have had less. They borrowed and used credit cards, but she said, "My kids are small and I need this help now. I may have the money in fifteen years if I save it, but then I won't need her." At the end of each day there was less stress for her and her husband. Today they are still very happily married, her children are succeeding brilliantly, and they are all very connected to each other.

I remember repeatedly turning away wonderful opportunities to see the world when I was in graduate school because I felt it was irresponsible, and I didn't have the money. I thought I shouldn't be taking a break from writing my thesis; I didn't want people to think I was irresponsible, and I was so wedded to my status as a starving student that I didn't take advantage of these opportunities. Ironically, as I went through my own journey, grew older, and learned to trust my gut, I would often embrace the fact that life is short, and somehow the bills would get paid. That kind of thinking has landed me on some low-budget, extraordinary adventures to Tibet, Peru, Greece, Italy, Spain, and other parts of the world. My spider senses told me the time was now, and a lifetime of experience reminded me that the bills eventually get paid. Today is the rainy day. I am not saying start spending frivolously, but I am saying that every so often you should lift up your head, trust your heart, stop living for a day down the road, and take a fiscal leap.

Interestingly, this lesson has fascinating implications for the dinner table. Many times we apply this thinking to eating. Instead of saving our pennies for a rainy day, we save our calories for dinner. It doesn't work that way. Yes, at a fundamental level there are 3,500 calories in a pound. However, most people who starve themselves all day so they can eat more at night lose their ability to be effective counters. Bingeing often follows a day of deprivation, and we end up eating in a dysregulated way, with the rationalization that "I didn't eat a thing all day."

In addition, eating the majority of your calories in one sitting, especially later in the day, is not optimal from a metabolic standpoint, and the overly acute sense of hunger can throw off all of our spider senses around hunger, fullness, and portion size. Saving and eating are all about balance. Be prudent, but not austere. Saving all your money for a day down the road and not living now is a bit much, just like subsisting solely on steamed vegetables and never having that occasional (but well-portioned) indulgence could make for a rather bland life.

New rule: Sometimes you need to act like the rainy day has arrived.

"Pride Goeth before a Fall"

Women take this one too seriously: Don't toot your own horn, whether it's in the workplace or at home. I am on an interesting e-mail list of women psychologists, and it is fascinating to observe how difficult it is for women to boast about their accomplishments, or even mention them. Women are taught almost in utero to not be prideful, and many an old wives' tale reflects on the fact that a prideful woman does not marriage material make. Many of us were raised on the evil eye—say something good about yourself, or even if someone else says something good about you, and that evil eye will seek you out and you're toast.

You can't give someone a swelled head by telling them they are good. Instead, it will actually build up their sense of efficacy, confidence, trust in their spider senses, and success. When you do something good and share such news appropriately, or if you feel good about your abilities and communicate that, your confidence and self-assuredness increases, as does your likelihood of a successful outcome. Denial of "pride" is at the core of so many difficulties with having a sense of self-worth and self-efficacy. Own your accomplishments. Learn how to share them appropriately and welcome hearing similar statements from others. Often we silence others' good news because it makes us take harsher measure of ourselves.

The old saying "Pride goeth before a fall" reflects false pride with little substantiation. It was Aesop's take on narcissism. But we have co-opted it, and any level of confidence is often viewed with suspicion. When we utter statements of pride, they are often followed by a pregnant pause as we wait for the other shoe to drop. Spider senses will usually allow you to accurately put those statements out at the right times.

New rule: Perhaps pride begets success and goeth before a triumph.

Dessert Is Bad for You

Everything is bad for you when you are consuming it for the wrong reason, and that includes dessert (or other kinds of food), or love. Most of us were taught that vegetables and other healthy foods are good, while dessert, cookies, and ice cream are bad. Our Calvinist culture tends to believe that pleasure is bad and struggle is good. Fun: bad. Hard work: good. Grilled chicken: good. Ice cream sundae: bad. Yet we are a country of pleasure junkies. Just turn on the TV and we're all scrambling to get our fix of sex, junk foods, and gambling. But pleasure and joy shouldn't be a fix; instead, they should be a regular a part of life just as work, or struggle, is. As a result, when we are finally faced with pleasure, we often don't know how to regulate it, and those feelings of being out of control can sometimes lead us to either push it out or become somewhat secretive about it. Shame is very much at the core of eating disorders and substance abuse, and many other disorders where regulation is thrown off.

Dessert shouldn't be misused as a reward or prize, or as something forbidden. Doing so gives it power, a bit like money. Our spider senses get thrown because we don't just view dessert as a food, but rather as something that means so many other things to us, and has since we were children. We've viewed a sweet treat as a celebration, an escape, a joy, or a cure for sadness for so long that we don't always trust our gut to let us have a little bit and move on, because it means so much more than just something that tastes good in that moment. Pleasure is good. Dessert is good. Fruits are good. It's about balance.

New rule: Pleasure and dessert should be a regular part of your life, not just a rare treat.

Clean Your Plate

Since more than half of Americans clean their plates at the table, I think it's fair to say that this is the most classic and damaging food lesson: The clean-plate club is really at the heart of this book. I learned this lesson as a child and then struggled with it right into my forties. If you can't walk away from a plate of food when you are full, how are you going to be able to walk away from a relationship or marriage when it's done, or a job when it's wrong? We were taught to put our heads down and eat ourselves numb, and then one day we find ourselves putting our heads down and living ourselves numb. Remember, the plate you usually clean is often filled by someone else. The tales we were taught played on guilt: If you don't eat that you are ungrateful; others are starving in the world; you are wasting food. Take that lesson and think about how it applies to your life: By taking a job for granted, you may think you are ungrateful; by leaving a marriage, you are letting down your entire family.

I think the clean-plate concept we were raised on is a disaster. I think we should encourage our children to join the dirty-plate club instead—to stop eating when they are full, even if there is food left on the plate, and to understand that it's okay to walk away. Once upon a time, as recently as forty or fifty years ago in this country, food was relatively expensive, many families struggled, and few folks regularly ate out. Portion sizes have gone up 30 percent in the last thirty years but our appetites have not.

Nonetheless,obesity statistics have skyrocketed along with these increases in portion sizes. Food is no longer a rare commodity—though in our society healthy food is. I understand waste is looked poorly upon, and I try to economize and stretch my pennies just like you. But eating food on your plate just because it is there has much more costly implications than the price of the fifteen noodles and quarter of a piece of burger you toss into the garbage can: obesity and being overweight can cost you and your children their lives. These costs can and will include medication and doctor's bills and the toll on your psyche—all of which is more expensive than the food you're tossing. *Wasting food in the short-term may buy you health in the long-term.* I will teach you about gatekeeping, so that when you are buying groceries or making meals you can attempt to limit waste. But when someone else is filling that plate, let go of your old scripts about waste if you want to get control of your waist.

New rule: When you're full, walk away and join the dirty-plate club.

DIRTY-PLATE CHALLENGES

We don't leave food on the plate because:
- we feel guilty,
- we are wasting money,
- there are starving children elsewhere, or
- it's an insult to the chef.

THE WHY

These new rules are a retelling of old ones, and require you to cast aside simple teachings and listen to your inner voice. However, the original golden rules are in your DNA and almost feel like reflexes. This isn't just an internal shift; it's an external shift, a new way of being in the world.

These rules scramble our spider senses because we were taught them at such a young age. They're mantras that often force us to deny our instincts. We started learning a lot of them for the sake of safety: Don't run in the streets, be home before dark, don't talk to strangers. Interestingly, many kids would have found the safety stories on the basis of instinct and spider senses. The bulk of these golden rules are rules of order—a way to make the lives of the rule-makers easier. The golden rules and fairy tales actually channel the stakeholders and play upon our fears to tamp down our spider senses. The golden rules are almost reflexive spider-sense scramblers because their roots run deep. When our spider senses steer us away from conventional wisdom, the golden rules can throw us.

THE NOW

STEP 1:
Take out your journal and create a section called "Golden Rules." Try to figure out the golden rules that most impact you and make a note of them. This could involve remembering stories told to you by grand-parents, stories you read, parables shared as part of your religious com-munity as a child, or even stories you choose to read to your children now. You can simply make a note of the title of the story or write a brief summary of it. Also reflect on social, cultural, or religious rules of order you were raised on.

STEP 2:
Make a note of how the golden rules you listed have impacted your life's decisions. Reflect on whether just relying on the golden rules—even if they made the outcome less than optimal—simply made the decision-making easier at that time. Sometimes the golden rules make things sim-ple right out of the gate and require us to take less responsibility, and that is why we often fall back on them. Think about some big-ticket decisions and then write down a few in your journal. What rules did you break, or abide by? What was the outcome in each case?

Your Life Is Not a Movie
While the golden rules came to us in childhood, we now know that they still have a *current* effect. That said, golden rules still come to us, albeit not as powerfully. Think about how you have been affected by films or television programs that you have recently seen. One of my favorite movie lines is from *Sleepless in Seattle,* where the best friend utters, "That's your

problem—the movies. You don't want to be in love, you want to be in love in a movie." It's a great line because many of us want the soft-scripted and unreasonable-ideal loves and lives depicted on the big screen.

Make a list of the movies, television shows, and books that influence you and your spider senses. Make a note of how they do this, and how they create the rules you want to live by. These books, films, and TV shows may also be driving a grandiose fantasy life; perhaps you aspire to live a lifestyle like that portrayed on a reality show, or stare agog at royal weddings. Think long and hard about this, because while you wait for some unrealistic fantasy, it's a bit like numbing yourself from real life.

On the other hand, these internalized messages may not all be bad, and they may be congruent with your spider senses. The key here is to be aware of how outside cultural influences shape you and your spider senses. Think about how these films, programs, and books are currently impacting your choices and how you think about your life.

A very fun add-on here is to have a film festival of your own where you bring together friends who share the film that has most influenced them and discuss why that is. How much have the actions of the characters in the film impacted your spider senses? Remind yourself that the characters are part of a script—and it is fiction. Not only may it give you tremendous insight into your friends, but it may also give them a new perception of you, and allow for all of you to discuss and reflect on how films and/or TV actually influence the choices you make now—good, bad, and indifferent.

Each day, before you make a decision, think about whether the golden rules are factoring in to your decision. Take a moment to breathe and let your spider senses flow, and determine whether you are making better decisions by not allowing golden rules—both new and old—to dictate your choices and actions when you know better.

CHECK-IN: GOLDEN RULES

Break one of your golden rules each day in a way that honors your spider senses. Leave a dirty plate, talk before you raise your hand, say hello to a stranger, take a chance, be proud of yourself and say it out loud. Don't just break rules to break rules, but trust your gut and your judgment. Make a mental note each day of how it turns out for you and how it feels afterwards.

As you complete your daily check-ins (or somewhat weekly check-ins) and think about choices, reflect on how your daily choices were affected by your golden rules. For example, did you offer to give someone a ride because it was the friendly good Girl Scout thing to do, but then it subsequently made you late and somewhat resentful?

CHAPTER 4

Conquering Fear

Fear makes come true that which one is afraid of.

—Viktor Frankl

Jill's mother's simultaneous fear of weight gain and fear of her daughter's burgeoning beauty set the tone in the household. The mother had frequent extramarital affairs, and the loud fights between her parents about these indiscretions filled the house with more fear. There was nowhere to escape from it. Being thin, slender, and blonde made it easy for Jill to meet men during adolescence and young adulthood, but fear about men's reactions to her beauty would often lead to eating. Jill's mother would chide her for not prettying herself up while attempting to compete with her. Over time, managing weight and fears about food led Jill to out-of-control binges and then bouts of vomiting. This binge-purge pattern would be punctuated by periods of restriction. Over time, the numbness that eating brought won out; it numbed anxiety, fear, exhaustion, and the demands of a grueling work schedule. When Jill reached 300 pounds, still as luminous as ever but carrying an unhealthy weight, it was time to start excavating through her story to get to the root of the fears and, ultimately, the eating. The pattern revealed itself: When the old fears and new fears ballooned—fears about family, fears about failure, fears about letting others down—the binges hit.

This patient's story brings home the point of fear because it illustrates the many places fear comes from. In her case, Jill's fears stemmed from watching her mother and her parents' relationships, along with anxiety about her own sexuality, about gaining—and losing—weight, and a general fear of food. In the midst of that, just picking up a cookie starts to feel like a horror film.

WHAT ARE YOU MOST AFRAID OF?

Before you read any further, grab your journal and make a list of things you're afraid of—anything at all. It is your private journal, so write it all down.

Take a look at what you wrote. Keep in mind that the most common fears are death, illness, infirmity, loss, poverty, and loneliness. These are fears that make a lot of sense; they're understandable. But fearing these things can put us at risk when, in our quest to avoid them, we make odd decisions.

Once we really give in to the common fears, we often start descending into other, more swampy fears: fear of not being able to take care of ourselves, fear of not being loved, fear of not being good enough, fear of things not working out, fear of taking chances, fear of change, fear of failure, fear of success, fear of growth, and fear of responsibility. So we construct lives that keep us from having to face these fears.

Many of these fears emerge around food—and fears about food, how to eat, what to eat, body image, and weight can lead to lifelong battles with food and eating. Fear is a killer when it comes to favorite foods: We fear being out of control, not having enough, and gaining weight from eating them. Sadly, this can lead us to behave badly in the presence of these foods.

The key is to learn to get beyond the fear, to overcome it, and to conquer it. When you have the upper hand at the table, you won't need to rely on stakeholders or prepackaged, robotic, one-size-fits-all meal plans.

WHY DO WE PANIC WHEN A PORTION IS SMALL?

I call this the "famine mentality." I was raised with this because my parents grew up in India at a time when food was scarce. Although their parents had enough, there was just enough, and all around them the impact of starvation was never far away. Food was sacred. If you believe there might not be enough, you worry. In such a setting, not being able to get food could induce feelings of panic and ultimately some strange relationships with food.

Perhaps attachment theory has some applicability to food and why small portion sizes can sometimes throw us when we are trying to manage our weight. People who are securely attached to food may not feel panicky when the food disappears; they may feel comfortable when food is placed in front of them, and have an easy, breezy relationship with food. People who are insecurely attached to food may feel scared that there will not be enough and genuinely upset when the food is gone; therefore, they may feel out of control when food is put in front of them. Most slender people I know who have never struggled with food don't even think about it; they eat, and when they're finished they stop thinking about it. Most people I know who struggle with food and weight ruminate about food all the time.

However, it's not always this linear. I have worked with many people who report that they were raised in homes with healthy rules around food: no clean-plate club, no tension at the table, parents who ate in a healthy manner. But in some cases they married into families with more-challenging paradigms about food. I worked with one client in particular who came from a family with very healthy eating patterns, who then married a man whose family was rather skewed about food. His parents were extremely controlling about expecting others to eat on their schedule, and would chastise her if she did not order the same quantities as others, or finish her food. She also noticed that her husband's pattern of eating involved a very large dinner after a long day of work, and that throughout her life with him, managing her weight remained a struggle. Ironically, the only time she reported being able to keep her weight at the level she wanted was when they had to live apart for a summer. She values her marriage and the relationships around her, so for her, finding a weight-management plan that can fit around the demands of her stakeholders has been no easy task.

UNDERSTANDING YOUR EATING ENVIRONMENTS AND APPROACHES

I still see around me parents who adhere to the call of the clean-plate club. My daughter Maya and I were once visiting with friends of the family, and we noticed that all of the children loaded up their own plates and sat down at the table. Maya didn't finish all of the food on her plate—not even close—and when she was done eating, she told me she was full. I told her that was fine, asked her to clear her plate, and sent her on her way. Interestingly, another child at the table observed this interaction. She has a father who is a charter member of the clean-plate club, at times tyrannical about the need to consume everything on the plate. She started chiding Maya about finishing all of the food on her plate. I warmly looked at the other child and said, "Actually, at our house we just stop when we are full. Next time, I hope Maya will be more mindful and put a little less on her plate." The other girl dutifully finished everything on her plate. I learned later that she has been struggling with her weight since she was about nine years old.

I grew up in a clean-plate family, and I feel strongly about the contribution of early environment or current environment to food-consumption patterns and fears about food. It is often easy to see how our current environment contributes to how we eat. Love handles are literally love handles (or unloved handles). Nobody can win here. People in relationships eat together; people who are single eat alone, or with friends and family. While some people report that once they got into a relationship they took on their partner's eating habits (usually to bad outcomes), you also may find yourself eating more regularly because of the greater likelihood of sitting down and having meals together. Neither group is free from emotional eating; a single person is just as likely as a partnered person to do so. Your current relationship status will impact your *current eating environments.*

Past environments are trickier. Let me tell you what dinnertime in my childhood home was like. It was tension upon tension. Fear of eating inadequately and speaking incorrectly was always present. My parents had a deprivation mentality in part due to their own histories in India, and "wasting" was not an option. Even the vocabulary of eating was pathologic.

- "Show your mom you love her and eat that curry."
- "Show me you love me and eat this dessert."
- "Good girls eat all the food on their plate."
- "You are not leaving the table until you finish it."

This culminated in all kinds of disordered eating habits, such that when I was full, I would put more in my mouth, ask to be excused, and then spit it out in the bathroom, spit it out in napkins, and so on. At an early age, a feeling of fullness did not imply the end of a meal—the edict of another did. And I would engage in whatever trickery was necessary to get through the meal. Over time I just ate to please, and I must have pleased the heck out of them, because as you know, at my heaviest I tipped the scales at well over 200 pounds.

The rhythms of my own house here in Los Angeles, where I reside with my two daughters, are interesting. On a recent Sunday afternoon, I awoke before dawn to work on this book, and then had some fruit at my desk. My older daughter woke up and did her own thing, getting some fruit and yogurt. An hour later her younger sister awakened and was hungry. I sat with her, had some fruit and tea while she ate her breakfast, and enjoyed the conversation with her. The older one was hungry about an hour later, and then all three of us joined together—we didn't eat, we just sat with her. We wanted her company, but we did not feel compelled to eat just to be at the table with her. We all ate in an organic rhythm, honoring our bodies, listening to them, but still coming together. What could seem like "selfish" rhythms from the outside—not honoring "mealtimes"— actually was an attempt by me to teach my girls on an unstructured day to learn what hungry and full feel like, that even when they are not on the schedule of another, they can honor and enjoy each other's company.

Different eating approaches work for different people, and there is no single plan that fits all. Some people don't do well with grazing all day; they tend to overeat each time, make bad choices, and may over-consume. Some people don't do well with scheduled mealtimes. By and large, many of the current weight-loss plans, and even treatment plans for women with binge-eating disorder and bulimia nervosa, strongly recommend scheduled mealtimes that must be honored. The goal of this is to avoid the hungry feeling that can often lead to overeating, to ensure that a person feels sustained and has equal energy throughout the day.

I am sometimes leery of plans that require you to eat at certain times because it represents an outsourcing of spider senses, but that is when we need to take a step back. If your spider senses work better with a schedule, that's different. When we break down the science of willpower, this does make sense in some ways. The problem is that many of us do not have the luxury of set schedules. My work doesn't always allow for me to eat a carefully portioned meal at noon. I don't think there is a perfect solution; I think there is only *your* solution. If you know that grazing is a problem for you, that you have difficulty managing your portions, then your spider senses are telling you that. Honor those feelings and harness regular mealtimes that work for you. If someone tries to put you on a set mealtime plan that you know would be all but impossible for you, and you are able to tolerate grazing, respond to hunger cues, and honor your spider senses and walk away, then listen to yourself. Some of the first food exercises we will do in the food chapters relate to you learning what *full* feels like for you by eating slowly. Whatever "eating plan" you decide on, make sure that it involves honoring yourself and your rhythms.

These attachments, fears, and rhythms with food are set early; in many cases, the way we learn to relate to food is also how we learn to relate with our early caregivers.

THE SOURCE OF FEAR

Fear can emanate from many places. True fear and realistic anxiety are useful because they keep us out of trouble—like knowing to be aware and move to safety on a dark street when we hear footsteps. But beyond that, fear is often learned, and learning takes place in three major ways, the same way we learn how to eat, work, love, and live:

- It is reinforced.
- It is paired with something else.
- We watch other people live in fear.

Fear through Reinforcement

Reinforcement has a lot of bearing on why we eat the way we do. Reinforcement serves to keep a behavior in place and it works through reward. Reward a behavior and it is repeated. If a child does something we like and we give him a gold star, he will repeat the behavior. Fears can be reinforced by parents or teachers who gave us more attention, hugs, or comforting words when we expressed fear.

Reinforcement doesn't just relate to fear. Let's start at the beginning. A fundamental and defining reinforcement we received was in the smiles and "happies" from whomever was feeding us when we were infants. As kids, parents would be happy when we ate our food with gusto. Good work would be rewarded with cookies and sweets both at home and school.

You were such a good girl during your haircut; here's a lollipop. When your mom wanted to shut you up, in sheer exasperation she may have given you a cookie. And guess how you reinforce yourself now as an adult? Yes, that same cookie. Fears are reinforced the same way—when we expressed fear, we would get attention, and that would often keep it in place.

What about other areas of our lives? When a relationship works and works well, it is inherently reinforcing. You say good things to your partner, he or she says good things to you, and together, growth takes place. There are other reinforcements that keep relationships in place too, ranging from tax incentives to the support of stakeholders to regular sex (maybe?). But the reinforcement of fear is often what keeps relationships in place: the fear of being alone, dying alone, being left to take care of ourselves. And in life, we may work harder if we are rewarded (e.g., staying in a job if people praise us for doing so). Sometimes reinforcement can keep something authentic and real in place, and sometimes it may force us to stay in a lie.

UNIVERSAL FEARS

Albert Ellis, a psychologist and founder of Rational Emotive Therapy, talks about the twelve irrational beliefs that fuel most of our illogical behavior (see resources section for a list of the twelve beliefs). Many of these underlie the universal fears around the need to always be accepted, always be liked, always be competent, life not turning out the way we want, and the idea that there is a right solution to each problem. These irrational beliefs and the fears that underlie them can often catapult us to struggle with decisions and with simply engaging in the business of living.

When Fear Is Paired with Something Else

Classical conditioning emanated from the work of Ivan Pavlov—experiments that anyone who has ever taken an introductory psychology class remembers. A dog smells meat and salivates. A bell rings every time meat is presented, and over time, when the dog hears the bell, the dog salivates even when there is no meat present. I call it the food poisoning paradigm.

If you eat shrimp scampi once and throw up violently afterwards, you are not going to eat it again for a very long time, and the look and smell of it will turn your stomach for months (or years) to come.

Classical conditioning—pairing a neutral stimulus with an unlearned, reflexive one—is a powerful and efficient way to learn fear, and is considered the genesis of most phobias. Theorists like John Watson believed that we could condition a phobia of an innocuous object quite easily, and generalize it to similar objects. We are born relatively fearless of most things, but some things are hardwired; for example, sudden loud noises. So when that sudden loud noise is paired consistently with something that we shouldn't be afraid of, over time we develop a fear of it because of the noise that always accompanied it.

Sometimes these lessons are classically conditioned lessons at the childhood dinner table, and eating gets paired with anxiety. This can make food fraught with conflict from an early age. That doesn't mean we can't fight this, largely by *unconditioning* the original conditioning. But the more intensive the conditioning, the harder it is to break it. Sometimes just the smell of an apple pie can take us back to conflicted family holidays. We just need to "reeducate" our brains, reconstruct those memories, and make the apple pie in a new setting with a new story.

You can learn to recondition the meaning of the dining table, to re-render the meaning of food in your life. The best way to do this is to pair something that makes us anxious—for example, eating with certain people or family members—with relaxation. Take a moment before going into the situation and take some deep breaths. Focus on the relaxed feelings, and even in the midst of what may have been traditionally an anxiety-provoking or just plain scary meal experience, you can start associating the feeling of relaxation with that space. Are there foods that you associate with being out of control, like ice cream? Create a relaxed situation. Work on deep breathing, deeply inhaling, filling in your lungs, and then slowly exhaling. Prepare a small serving of that food, and while you are sitting with it, before you ever eat it, keep breathing slowly and deeply. Breathe in the presence of it, put it in your mouth, and savor it, remaining relaxed and staying focused on the relaxed feeling. You can't just do this once; it's necessary to do it several times, or each time you are in the situation. Over time you may be able to feel relaxed with those foods instead of experiencing the automatic feelings of fear and anxiety.

Watching Other People Live in Fear

Observing people is an efficient way of learning anything, especially fear. Think of the last time you were in a fearful situation: You likely looked around at how others were reacting, and if they were reacting fearfully, often your reaction would transition over to fear. We learn fearlessness the same way: by watching others. Thus, growing up with fearful parents begets fear. And in the bubble-wrapped culture of modern parenting, fearfulness has become endemic. At the dinner table a mother with fears of weight gain can communicate her fears of certain foods to a child, or a parent's fear about not having enough food can stimulate such fears in a child. Much of how we learn to function in our lives—in love, work, food, and play—was learned by watching others. And if we watched fearful models, that fear will carry over into all aspects of our lives.

FEARED FOOD MISTAKE: AVOIDING THEM ALTOGETHER

When we are afraid of something, we avoid it. That means everything, including food. If we feel like we can't control ourselves with a particular food and we are trying to lose weight, then that food feels scary and we avoid it. The problem is, we will be faced with that food again, and then what? How will we react? As a result many of us live and eat from a place of deprivation; we cut out the scary foods and things altogether. The problem is, this doesn't work. You need to invite the demons to the table and learn to eat with them.

Willpower can teach us a lot about fear. We think that by cutting out the scary stuff we have mastered fear. Nope. Willpower does not generate more willpower. In fact, the opposite is true. Research conducted by Roy Baumeister—a psychology professor at Florida State University, and a scholar who has contributed significantly to our understanding of willpower and decision-making—nicely points out that willpower is a finite resource. Once you start expending it, you start running out of it. So once you cut out a food group, ultimately you may end up wanting it more and more. Many people talk about how they are afraid of the many choices and foods they are faced with; by understanding how willpower works, you can become stronger instead of panicked in the face of these choices.

Roy Baumeister and his team conducted an interesting experiment where they brought research participants into the lab. Before coming in, one group was required to avoid temptations such as candies and sweets. This group had a harder time showing self-discipline or exertion. For example, they gave up more quickly on lab tasks such as math problems or a test of handgrip strength (a measure of effort, on which we tend to expend less energy when our willpower is depleted) when compared to the research participants who were allowed to indulge in the temptation of sweets.

Willpower does not generate more willpower. In fact, the opposite is true. Willpower is a finite resource. Once you start expending it, you start running out of it.

We live in a society where self-control is over-valued at some level. We value people who don't eat very much, who are ultra-organized, who don't always show their emotions. The problem is that you have a finite well of self-control to use throughout the day, and the more you rely on it, the less of it you will have. Research by Wilhelm Hofmann, an assistant professor of psychology at the University of Chicago, suggests that we spend a considerable amount of time each day in a state of "desire," wanting to eat treats, fool around on the computer, kick it with friends, tell someone off, have sex, or check Facebook. The more you resist these desires, the more vulnerable you become to caving in to the next temptation that comes along.

Baumeister and his colleague Jean Twenge also did a study on the topic of "decision fatigue." Given more options or more to choose from, participants show less self-regulation. This may be why you feel out of control when you go to an all-you-can-eat buffet with lots of choices. But choice is good . . . right? Not necessarily. If you are buying a house, making decisions about an event, or planning a vacation, after a while, you get burned out and capitulate. The overwhelming number of choices leaves you exhausted and incapable of making smart decisions, or any decisions for that matter.

There is often a lot of hypothesizing about why our ancestors had better willpower than we do today. They probably did. According to

Baumeister, they just didn't have as many choices to make or options to act on. The downside was that they were often restricted in what they could do with their lives; the upside was that they were less likely to succumb to temptations and overdo it (and there were fewer temptations out there). These unlimited choices doom so many of us not only when it comes to weight, but also other life choices. It's why we carry fifty extra pounds and have twenty pairs of black shoes we don't wear.

The fact is, we live in a world full of choices, and choices can be overwhelming, if not downright scary. It's hard to live in this world and limit our options, but we can do it in some settings. Take control whenever you can. Avoid buffets; they may seem like more bang for your buck, but it's just too easy to overdo it.

It's easy to get overwhelmed and depleted and start making bad choices. On days when you have to make a big-ticket decision, minimize other choices—either ask other people to step in, or just make the day less complex by not putting yourself in the line of fire (for example, on such days avoid shopping, making choices at a restaurant, or making a decision for a group, such as what movie you are going to see). Focus on the big decision that needs to be made that day and don't clutter the landscape with lots of other choices. If you regularly face many choices in your work or as a parent, then find ways to fast-track other decision-making tasks. Purchase the goodies for the bake sale or potluck; don't go to the mall for the gift, order a gift card online; let someone else pick the movie or restaurant.

Let's compare these food fears to unrequited love. Think about that person you wanted to be with, but with whom you couldn't or shouldn't have a relationship. You thought about him *all* the time, and then when you were with him, you felt out of control, because you didn't know when you would see him again. Needless to say, the relationship probably didn't go well. That wild, crazy lover is forbidden fruit, and you often ruin yourself in the pursuit of it. Did you see *Like Crazy?* It was a wonderful movie about the angst of two young lovers who spent years trying to be together, but they were hampered by one's inability to get a visa to move to the United States. In the end, years later, after all the desire and desperation, they finally got together and the feeling of "What now?" overwhelmed the closing scene. My guess: They broke up a few months later.

If you want to manage those forbidden and scary foods, here's the best suggestion: Engage in the greatest romance killer of all and marry them. Marry them? Yes; make a commitment to them, one that you have to adhere to day in and day out. Until it gets dull. And you grow to appreciate them, but find that you don't need to gorge on them. Give yourself a daily prescription of the "scary" food. I had one patient to whom I gave a prescription to eat a 100-calorie candy bar sold by a local grocery store at 3 p.m. each day. According to her, chocolate was her weakness, and she often felt out of control after entirely avoiding it for many weeks. These 100-calorie bars were individually wrapped, tasty, and manageable, and they satisfied her. After a few weeks, the 100-calorie bar lost its luster, and chocolate stopped feeling like such an out-of-control temptation. After about two weeks, of required chocolate she reported not caring about whether or not she ate the chocolate, and found that she no longer felt out of control with it.

Sexy Food and Fear

I personally have a list of foods that are my food-porn go-to's. They are lasagna, hamburgers, pizza, pasta, grilled cheese, and sandwiches on good bread. I daydream about these foods, and at some level I am afraid of them because I do feel out of control with their seductive powers. So now I invite them in. Once a week, one of these foods comes in, in a manageable portion with a large salad or steamed vegetables on the side. Because I know they are coming they don't scare me. I look forward to them, and welcome them in like an occasional guest. When I attempted to kick them out altogether, things always got a bit out of control. Now when I'm around lasagna, I'm able to consume it without the crazy passion and fear.

Donuts are another big, scary, forbidden porn food for me. Back in the day, when I really struggled with my weight, I ate two or three a day without thinking about it. The pink and orange letters of Dunkin' Donuts are as classically conditioned for me as any Pavlovian stimulus. When I was in the Atlanta airport recently, the pink sign beckoned, I was hungry, and I went in. I wanted a bite. Just a bite. So I had my bite and threw it out. I didn't let fear lead me to binge on it or avoid it. I felt like I showed that donut who was boss. Somehow not buying it felt too deprivational, while eating it all felt excessive. I was alone, which made it easier, because trying to throw it out under the watchful eyes of another would have left me feeling like I would have to rationalize this bizarre decision.

WHY DOES FEAR MAKE US EAT MORE OFTEN THAN WE SHOULD . . . OR NOT EAT?

Remember, fear scrambles and all but shuts down our spider senses; it's the equivalent of taking a cell phone into the sixth-floor basement of a parking garage. And as such, our ability to know we are full or hungry gets thrown, and we become vulnerable to signals that have nothing to do with hunger or fullness.

Fear can certainly contribute to overeating in a number of ways: We overeat to numb the fear, to avoid the thing we fear, to numb our sense of fullness, and to numb our fears of feeling hungry, empty, letting others down, and breaking childhood rules.

Fear can also contribute to undereating: to avoid weight gain, or to exert control in a situation where other modes of communication may feel too frightening. In many eating disorders, fear of gaining weight and fear of being overweight can lead to dangerous behaviors, and it is just as much a denial of spider senses as overeating.

FEAR AND FOOD

WHY FEAR RESULTS IN OVEREATING:
- Fear of feeling hungry or empty
- Avoid feelings we fear
- Fear of letting other people down
- To numb fears
- Fear of breaking rules

WHY FEAR RESULTS IN UNDEREATING:
- Fear of being out of control
- Fear of being overweight or gaining weight
- "Safer" way to communicate needs or exert control

FEAR AND SCRIPTS

A last word here on where fears hold some of their greatest power—on a future that has not yet been realized. We use scripts to organize our lives, often to disastrous results. Scripts can often force us into the story we expect will happen rather than the one unfolding in front of us. Given that fear is a powerful editor, it can take our scripts to dark places. *If I eat that I will get fat, and no one will ever love me. I will always be overweight. That man is going to hurt me, so why bother even opening myself up to him?* That anticipated ending can lead us to behave accordingly—whether it's eating mindlessly or holding back in a new relationship. People can be loved at any weight. And yes, he may hurt you. But to hold back because of something that might happen is like putting a seat belt on your soul and spider senses. Let the story unfold; stop trying to write it, and stop skipping to the last page. Give life, your spider senses, and yourself a chance. Broken hearts heal, but regret never dissipates.

THE WHY

Fears can shut us down and lead us to stop listening to ourselves. Fears gum up our works, silence our spider senses, and are usually met with avoidance. People eat to avoid feelings. People have fears about foods and eating situations that can make it challenging to eat in those situations. Fears also extend into our relationships. Fear can be like superglue in a relationship. For example, people who are terrified of being alone may cling to a broken relationship with an iron grip for fear it will be their last chance at love ever. Fear can also give our stakeholders even more power, because fear of losing them, or even fear of pleasing them, can lead to some absolute denial of our spider senses in all situations.

The best way to choose the wrong door, or never even open the door, is to let fear run the show. When you reflect on any big-ticket decision you have made on the basis of fear and anxiety, you can almost guarantee you made the wrong decision.

We give fear its power—and that means we can take it back. Fear drives lots of bad behaviors, largely through avoidance. For most of us, fear is not a comfortable feeling, so we will do just about anything to avoid it. It is a bit paradoxical; instead of fear leading us to walk away, sometimes it leads us to sticking around so we don't break any rules.

THE NOW

This exercise will require going back to what you did at the beginning of the chapter. Look at those fears you listed. Next to each fear, I want you to indicate what realms of your life it has impacted. Eating? Relationships? Work? School? Parenting? Other habits, such as spending or smoking? Ideally you will elaborate on this and explain how a given fear influenced something like eating. By understanding why a certain fear affects your behavior, you are better able to pay attention, monitor, and fix it.

How can we minimize the influence of fear? First of all, know what your fears are. You already did this by listing them. Second, once you've identified your pressure points of fear and you're facing a big decision, pay careful attention to how that fear could thwart your decision. Monitor and remain aware of *what you want,* so you can balance that against fear.

Third, face your fears. Make a catastrophe list. What would happen if the fears were realized? What if you were abandoned at the altar—what would that mean? Lifelong humiliation? Death? Terminal illness? By taking it to an absurd conclusion, and then slowly pedaling back, the fears are less likely to own you.

You may have lots of fears that have affected you throughout your life, but I want you to isolate those that imprison you and continue to have an impact on your behavior today. Each day this week, or as many days as possible, write down how fears are influencing your behavior. As you think about the Now, think about fears this way:

- What settings bring out fear—and how do they affect your spider senses?

- Which people bring out fear—and how do they weaken your spider senses?

- What tasks bring out fear—and how do they damage your spider senses?

- When you are scared, what behaviors do you turn to?

- When you are scared, how do you eat?

- What do you eat when you're afraid?

- How much do you eat when you're afraid?

Reflect on your answers and start thinking about how you can modify those settings, people, and tasks to make them less fearful. (Deep breathing? Communication? Relaxing? Self-talk?)

Look at those eating patterns and think about how you can face those fears differently. See if you find other substitute activities for fear. Make a list of five activities that you enjoy that are not eating to use when you are fearful. (Working out at the gym? Walking? Reading? Watching TV? Calling a friend?)

CHECK-IN: FEAR

Reflect on how a fear impacted your behavior and/or eating today. Think of a new way you can tackle that fear. For example, you may be afraid of letting down a friend by not giving her a ride, even though you know it would require lots of time you don't have that day. Think of another way to handle this fear and change your communication. If you need to role-play, practice telling your friend that you can't give her a ride today and tolerating the discomfort of telling her something she does not want to hear. This check-in is about practicing an alternate way to respond to fear each day.

CHAPTER 5

Gatekeeping

It is easier to stay out than to get out.

—Mark Twain

For a person who is struggling with weight management and weight loss, going to a restaurant is like mortal combat. I imagine it like some kind of video game—breadbasket hurtling at your head, appetizers being fired at you, large portions, big plates, and dessert. Eating out often is one of the things that contributes to weight gain. Restaurants tend to use richer ingredients and bigger portions than we do at home. The decisions begin the moment you sit down: Drink? Bread? Butter with that bread? What would you like to start with—appetizer or entree? And then for the pornographic finish, allow us to leave you a dessert menu to tantalize you, even though you just told us you don't want any. I remember frequently dining out with an old friend who would be embarrassed by just ordering an appetizer, and even apologize for it, despite the fact that in most restaurants an appetizer is in excess of a normal-size meal.

Within a sixty-minute meal we are faced with about ten decisions regarding food, and have to make healthy choices in the midst of a minefield. There are yummy smells, bread close enough to grab, and that frequent feeling that you are "owed" the fettuccine Alfredo because you had a bad day. And of course, there's the desire to please your waiter. Each choice is a gatekeeping opportunity: to not order too much; to order what you want, not what your friends want; to order for the right reasons; to eat a healthy quantity; and you have to do this in a context where you are feeling pressured by your fellow diners. And that's just one meal.

If you make good choices from the outset, you don't have to fix a bad decision down the road. That is gatekeeping. Imagine how gatekeeping jumps from the dinner table and into all areas of your life.

One of the best uses of our spider senses is to stop ourselves from entering bad situations in the first place. By trusting our spider senses, we become better gatekeepers. Many big-ticket decisions that involve entering into a long-term commitment are influenced by the voices of other people rather than our own instincts, and yet we are the ones stuck in the situation once we enter it.

That's where gatekeeping factors in. It is the most efficient way of using our spider senses because it stops us from entering bad situations at the outset. Getting out is always more difficult than getting in. Prevention is easier than the cure. Gatekeeping is about how much food we put on our plates, because once it's on our plates, we feel compelled to finish it, and the world expects us to finish it. So whether it's portion control, or walking away from the wrong partner before you say "I do," or not taking a bad job, you need to use your spider senses to gatekeep the decisions in your life. Whether you are on the cusp of a major decision or need help using spider senses in future decision-making, gatekeeping can protect you and the people around you from wasting time, emotional energy, and resources. Good gatekeeping then becomes a habit that results in keeping the toxic stuff out and allowing growth in.

Remember that spider senses are impacted by stakeholders, golden rules, and fears—and because gatekeeping can and should be impacted by spider senses, so too can gatekeeping get thrown by all of these things. Our stakeholders are a powerful influence in the kinds of decisions we make, including what we order and how much food we put on our plates. In a restaurant, even the chef and the wait staff are stakeholders. They have no idea how hungry you are, but they do know that if they don't give you enough, you may not come back. If you like their food, they feel good about their jobs and perhaps themselves. Golden rules such as "happily ever after" and the various scripts reinforced by the golden rules can lead us to ignore our spider senses when we are faced with new decisions. And fear may be the biggest gatekeeping killer of all: Our fears of everything—failure, success, letting other people down, or in the case of our plates, feeling out of control with food—can lead us to make suboptimal choices on the way in.

THE BRAIN-BODY CONNECTION

In 1994 Antonio Damasio wrote the groundbreaking book *Descartes' Error: Emotion, Reason, and the Human Brain,* in which he lays out a theory called the somatic marker hypothesis. It is an elegant model that cuts to the quick of understanding how we make decisions, and it has clear implications for gatekeeping. The somatic marker hypothesis says that our bodies, which are a large driving force behind our spider senses, work in cooperation with our thoughts and logic. Very simply, we cannot separate the two, which is in contrast to the idea that brain and body function independently. We are also not computers: We cannot apply steely logic to all that we do, try as we sometimes might. Life does not allow us the luxury of creating a lengthy pros and cons list for every decision we make, because frankly, it's too time-consuming, and it doesn't always work, especially for emotional decisions like choosing a life partner. The somatic marker hypothesis suggests that our gut instincts make us efficient by knocking out lots of options right away, allowing us to apply some logic to the options that remain when we make a decision. The challenge then becomes the fact that these somatic markers have developed within a context of culture, society, family, and learning. And there's the rub: Not all of these factors, including culture, society, and family, take us where we want to go—and yet in their fashion they drive our instincts / somatic markers.

A key element of Damasio's work is the issue of learning. Since the day we are born, we learn with a vengeance. The brains of children are electrically wired sponges that absorb everything—good, bad, and indifferent. That learning gets paired with emotions and physiological responses, and over time we pair those "feelings" with what seem to be rational decisions. We learn to do this through experience. So when we make certain kinds of decisions, we will have a certain bodily reaction and a certain set of emotions, and over time the choices and feelings become connected.

Here is an example: Perhaps mealtimes for you as a child were a time of anxiety, lots of fighting, and conflict. If you didn't eat everything on your plate, you knew anger from your parents would follow, and that would often leave you with a pit in your stomach. So over time, the dots connected between mealtime choices, feeling anxious, and the racing heart and sweaty palms at those times. So cleaning your plate became automatic, perhaps a way of avoiding the anxiety that mealtimes bring, and as such, it felt like a choice—even when it wasn't. Whether it's good or bad decisions, the pairing of bodily sensations and feelings can fast-track our decision-making. Our brains and bodies cooperate with the results of that experience, and bodily feelings, brain responses, and decision-making all occur in a beautifully orchestrated dance.

Where this can get tricky is that some of this learning—in fact, most of it—occurs within a societal context where we are liberally influenced by stakeholders and the world around us. At some level this is a necessity, since this is how we learn right from wrong, the rules and morals of a society. But it also means that our bodies, emotions, and minds are mired in the lessons of others—and to that degree, at some level our spider senses do have our stakeholders' fingerprints all over them. Yet, you know that many times in your own life, the thing that is right for you, instinctually, may be at odds with what your stakeholders want for you, even though they were the ones who taught you those lessons in the first place.

GATEKEEPING AND LONG-TERM DECISIONS

Gatekeeping is also influenced by the difficult act of balancing both long- and short-term decisions. One of our big struggles in making any decision—in essence, in knowing when to quit, walk away, and leave the plate—is balancing the long and the short term. We know how we feel now, but it's harder to determine how we will feel down the road. Psychologist Daniel Gilbert beautifully addresses this tricky balancing act in his analysis of future decision-making. He basically argues that we are not particularly accurate when we attempt to predict our own futures, and the rosy futures we predict for ourselves are biased by our assumptions, attributions, and skewed imagination about what the future may actually hold.

People tend to have more difficulty listening to others when it relates to their future. Not long ago I had lunch with a colleague who had recently had a baby. When she was pregnant, I had warned her that returning to the university after her maternity leave would be difficult, based on my own experience. She smiled politely at the time, but after she returned to work, she looked at me wide-eyed and exhausted and said, "This is really hard." I reminded her that I had predicted it would be tough, and she said, "I remember—but I just thought it would be different for me."

Gilbert argues that that the best source of information about our futures is other people's experiences, especially those currently living the future we want to have for ourselves. For example, if you want to know what your life will look like when you have a five-year-old child, don't imagine it; instead, talk to someone who has a five-year-old, or offer to take care of that child for the day.

Thus, when we gatekeep, we are trying to do two things at the same time. We want to balance both short- and long-term outcomes on the basis of experience and instinct. But since we aren't very good at accurately predicting our own futures, and our spider senses tend to get mangled by the webs of stakeholders, golden rules, and fear, we can instead make some really bad decisions initially. And many times we make these rather important decisions cavalierly, thinking we can simply fix them down the road.

Gatekeeping, or good front-end decision-making, takes place in the midst of this juggling of potential outcomes. For example, a young person named Wendy is deciding on a new job. Two offers come

We want to balance both short- and long-term outcomes on the basis of experience and instinct. But since we aren't very good at accurately predicting our own futures, and our spider senses tend to get derailed by the webs of stakeholders, golden rules, and fear, we can instead make some really bad decisions initially. And many times we make these rather important decisions cavalierly, thinking we can simply fix them down the road.

in: The first holds less opportunity for growth but is close to home, a boy-friend, and parents who don't want her to move too far away. The second offer, the job that feels "right," is on the other side of the country, far away from anyone she knows and likely to result in the end of her relationship with the boyfriend. Wendy not only has to weigh all the opinions, wants, and needs of her stakeholders, but she also has to address her fears, what she has been told is "right" since she was a child, and the long- and short-term implications. The short-term implications are clear: Staying local is easy, she gets to keep her life as usual, and there is little risk. The long-term implications are less known, but it's clear that the faraway job has better prospects—along with the likelihood that she'll lose her boyfriend and anger her parents. And that is frightening.

This is where spider senses become critical. Wendy doesn't have a crystal ball. She could talk to people who have experienced similar situations to see how things panned out for them, but ultimately, the only absolute certainty is what she instinctively knows is right for her. And that conviction would likely lead to the best possible gatekeeping situation. It also fosters taking responsibility for her own life.

Gatekeeping in this case not only has implications for her present, but also for her future. By heeding her spider senses, Wendy may have to work through an initial burst of discomfort and anxiety, but she is also likely creating a future that is more congruent with what she inherently knows is right. By ignoring her gatekeeping spider senses, she may find herself with a heap of regret and grow to resent her stakeholders. While in the short term it seems as though good gatekeeping could lead to estrangement between Wendy and her stakeholders, it is quite likely that sticking around could result in a brewing resentment that in the long run would be far more damaging to these close ties, and to her career prospects, than if she took the faraway job in the first place.

It is so easy to blame bad gatekeeping on others if we feel overly swayed by them. But if we honor ourselves, even if there is short-term sacrifice, our ownership of these decisions makes us more steadfast, and sets us on a course of taking responsibility and making bolder decisions.

The prevailing scientific wisdom says that we do honor our spider senses when we make decisions, but do we ever realize how aware we are of the things that influence us as we make these decisions—namely, the influences of our stakeholders, the golden rules, and fear? Even when we think we are following our gut instincts, those instincts are still shaped by the larger world. For example, our image of the "right person" for us romantically is actually a patchwork of a million messages from the world, our parents, and our cultures. That perfect mate will be in part what we think our parents want, what society tells us is attractive, what our childhood storybooks told us Prince (or Princess) Charming is all about, and the person who protects us from our fears (or plays into them) and who makes us feel safe. And some of those things do matter to us, so even our gut instincts aren't entirely ours.

But the question then remains: How much are we choosing on the basis of gut instincts that are shaped by the world, and how much are we choosing to please others, silence the voices around us, and cave in to our fears? Interestingly, when it comes to our gut, the one thing we are unable to do is listen to it. And this isn't just about the big-ticket decisions, such as choosing a life partner or a career. This is about a lifetime of gatekeeping at the table: Weight gain, weight loss, and weight management are all about the culmination of decisions over time.

GATEKEEPING AND OUR SPIDER SENSES

The following anecdote illustrates how your gatekeeping skills, whether ordering at a restaurant or choosing a mate, can benefit from listening to your spider senses. This is the tale of a man who had an important job, a large house, expensive cars, luxurious vacations, a beautiful wife, and two kids in private school. From the outside his life was great, and, in fact, enviable. It seemed he had everything he wanted. But in this guy's head, he had come to the realization that his marriage was over. He had had multiple affairs, including cheating on the women he was having affairs with. He had wanted to stay in the marriage for the sake of the children, until they were older. In his mind, he was doing the right thing. He made the decision to stick it out until his children moved out and then he would live the life he'd always wanted to live. He and his wife were no longer growing together, and their relationship had become disconnected. They tried the usual paths to fixing it—marriage counseling, working on communication. But he was done. Still, he stayed.

Unfortunately, one of his affairs was with a coworker, a move that breached his company's code of ethics. He was consequently fired, and at the same time the economy tanked. He lost the big house and all the goodies on which he'd spent his fortune over the years. He declared bankruptcy. His wife's psychological health suffered. There was massive collateral damage.

If this guy had just been true to himself, he would have ended his marriage in a timelier manner. Yes, his wife may have been devastated, but the type of psychological problems she suffered may not have been as pronounced, and his children would not have been exposed to nearly as much contention. Instead of trusting his spider senses and walking away when he was done, he thought he could keep stuffing himself.

When he looks back at the whole picture now, he realizes he got married too young, and for the wrong reasons. He hadn't used good gatekeeping early on in the relationship, and when he finally started to consider making a better decision about his life and that of his family, it was too late. The stakes were far too high, and the damage that came in the wake of the late decision, devastating.

So how did he get there, to that place called "too late"? Could it all have been avoided? Perhaps. When he reflects back, there were external reasons for forcing the marriage issue. Geographic and financial factors pushed their hand, and in the nearsightedness of youth, he asked his beautiful young girlfriend to marry him. As a young man would, he turned to his family for advice, and their guidance was consistent with the societal party line; her family was even less useful, and despite his spider senses telling him marriage was likely a foolhardy gamble, he ignored it all. "I will be different," he thought. "It will all work out; after all, we're in love. . . ."

Famous last words.

GATEKEEPING AND OUR STAKEHOLDERS

When you think about gatekeeping, keep in mind that making decisions in a vacuum is unrealistic, and that stakeholders do matter. Now, obviously, some integration of expert advice into our decision-making process is not always a bad thing. Turning to a tax expert or financial planner for input on how to invest a sum of money, or a contractor about the viability of a structural improvement on a home purchase, is a different matter. But that's not who or what I'm talking about here. I'm talking about being aware of those with a stake in the game of your life, and those stakes are not always in your best interest. The trick then becomes balancing the voices of your stakeholders against what you know is best for you, and that's where gatekeeping becomes critical.

Here are some tips on how to manage the competing voices of your stakeholders and your spider senses when you stand at the doorway of a big decision. These are ways to fine-tune your gatekeeping skills:

- Before asking everyone and their brother for advice, take the time to sit with yourself and think hard about what you want.

- Think ahead about what you know about your stakeholders and what they are going to say. You know them better than you think, and if you prepare for their reactions, you won't be as blindsided.

- Practice the "rope-a-dope" technique. In the legendary "Rumble in the Jungle" boxing match (Muhammad Ali vs. George Foreman), Ali harnessed Foreman's energy and used it against him. In essence, Ali was able to take a stance that allowed him to withstand Foreman's pummeling while backed up against the ropes instead of dancing away from them. By withstanding the punches he exhausted his opponent, and then with one swift jab, it was good night George. Much like Sun Tzu argues in *The Art of War,* learn how your opponent fights, learn to defend against his attack with a goal of exhausting him, and then do what you need to do. By relying on your spider senses you can strengthen your resolve, protect yourself, use their energy against your stakeholders, and let them exhaust themselves. Even they will get tired of listening to themselves as you listen, acknowledge, smile, and ultimately do what is right for you.

- Bring some objective sources in, if possible, and ask someone who has some experience with your situation for some guidance. If you want to know what it's like to live in Oregon, ask someone who lives in Oregon. If you want to know what it's like to adopt a child from another country, ask someone who has done it.

HOW TO FILL YOUR OWN PLATE IN THE FIRST PLACE

Let's put some of these gatekeeping techniques into practice as they apply to eating. If you put the right amount of food on your plate to begin with, you give yourself exactly what you need to enjoy your meal, and you don't have to engage in an internal debate over how much is too much while you're in the middle of dinner, and at your weakest. If it's on the plate, you'll eat it for a variety of reasons: because it's there, to please the others around you, or to avoid the villainy of waste. You're more easily swayed at that point. But if you learn to use portion control when you fill your plate, I suspect you'll be satisfied and won't eat for the wrong reasons. Remember, it's not always you who fills your plate; sometimes other people fill our plates for us—literally—at restaurants, or when you're having dinner at a friend's house. There are some tricks you can employ when you're eating to really help you gatekeep your plate at the outset:

Use smaller plates. Don't get lost in the parlor trick that certain-colored plates will lead you to eat more or less. If you can't put as much food on the plate, simple logistics will stop you.

Don't put platters of food on the table; instead, fill your plate in the kitchen, step away from the food, and sit down with your portioned meal.

Don't go to the kitchen for seconds.

Restaurants

Order an appetizer and a salad rather than an entree, or if you want the entree, ask if the restaurant offers a half portion or divide the full portion in half immediately and ask them to take away the other half. This messes with a lot of people's heads because they fret about the fact that they paid for all of it. You actually paid for the ambience, for someone else to cook for you and clean your dishes, and for the electricity in the restaurant. If you eat enough to fill you up, then you got your money's worth.

Leave your leftovers at the restaurant.

Choose restaurants wisely; use your gatekeeping skills to select restaurants that offer healthier options. The choices on the menu will be harder to navigate once you're at the table feeling hungry and tempted.

Dinner Parties

Finishing everything on your plate can get tricky when you're at someone else's house and afraid of insulting the host by leaving food. Here are a few tips that can help you navigate these situations smoothly:

Whenever possible, put your own food on your plate at someone else's house, so you can choose the right amount. Even offer to help in the kitchen to give you some control over this process. An added bonus: It makes you feel good to be helpful.

Get up and toss your own paper plate if it's a more casual setting; find a good break in the conversation and chuck it.

Don't assume the hostess cares how much you ate. Eat what you want, enjoy the conversation, and offer to clear the table (again, bonus points for helping).

If you are directly asked if you don't like the food because you didn't finish everything on your plate, *tell a white lie* ("I ate a late lunch"), or just *acknowledge being full* and directly state that the food was good. Don't apologize.

THE WHY

Gatekeeping is merely good front-end decision-making. At the table, it can simply be how much food you put on your plate or what you order in a restaurant. In life, it's about who you choose as a partner, the school you decide to attend, or the career you pursue. When we heed our spider senses at the beginning of a process and don't allow fear, golden rules, and stakeholders to run the show, we can make better decisions out of the gate instead of having to dismantle or defend them later. By monitoring your decision-making on a daily basis, you'll be better able to not only fill your plate more accurately, but also make better life decisions.

THE NOW

An exercise at the table:

In the next few weeks, practice gatekeeping at mealtimes. In the first week, just watch yourself; don't make any changes yet. Observe and ideally document how much you serve yourself, and whether it was easy to only eat what was on the plate and not go back for more. If you put too much on, was it more difficult to pass once it was in front of you? Are there patterns to your eating? Do you take larger quantities earlier in the day or later in the day? With other people? In certain settings? With certain foods?

Now do some real gatekeeping. If you notice a pattern of putting too much on your plate, fill your plate, take half of it off, then eat. Eat slowly and reflect on whether you are satisfied with this smaller portion.

Practice this in a restaurant. Order something and either split it with a friend or get rid of half of it, or whatever amount is needed to create a reasonable portion size, throwing out the rest (don't take it home with you). Again, ideally record this in your journal. Reflect first on what it was like to toss away the food or have it taken away. How did you feel? Wasteful? Anxious? In control? Then note whether or not you were satisfied after the meal.

Reflecting on past gatekeeping errors (or successes) right now may seem overwhelming, but it will provide important data for your ongoing decision-making. A pattern will likely emerge in which you find that you experienced more confidence (but perhaps more anxiety) in decisions where you listened to yourself—at the table, with your family, or in the office.

At the end of this exercise you will have some insight into the types of stakeholders, fears, and golden rules that impact your ability to gatekeep. This can inform you of your pressure points as you go into future gatekeeping situations.

Now, start paying attention. Start small at the table, and then apply it to larger decisions you are facing—major purchases, work, where to take a vacation. As you face decisions and gatekeeping, veer away from the usual pros and cons list and reflect instead on how fears, stakeholders, and golden rules are impacting this decision and your spider senses. You can then ensure that when you make choices, at least you are heeding these influences, and hopefully creating better gatekeeping moments every day.

CHECK-IN: GATEKEEPING

Now that you're aware of your ability to gatekeep, be conscious of how often you make decisions, big or small, in a day. Mentally rate the spider-sense-y inputs you are using in these decisions. Think about the gatekeeping decision(s), and then how much you trusted yourself, and, subsequently, your decision. Even more important, return to this gatekeeping section of your journal and look at how these decisions eventuated over time.

CHAPTER 6

Using Data Wisely

The other terror that scares us from self-trust is our con-
sistency; a reverence for our past act or word, because the
eyes of others have no other data for computing our orbit
than our past acts, and we are loath to disappoint them.
—Ralph Waldo Emerson

I realize you may not really know this or may have never even thought about it, but we live our lives by the scientific method. We never stop testing and learning. Whether we're aware of it or not, every day we collect data; we try out new things and discover that some work, and some don't. In theory, we should repeat the ones that do work and we should toss those that don't. If we had any sense we'd operate that way, but we know that's not always what happens. An elegant dance takes place between trusting our spider senses and collecting data. Striving to lose weight is a great example of this—we try diets and exercise, and yet find ourselves in the same place over and over again. This occurs because we often ignore our inner voices and eat things we don't like in ways that don't make sense.

We rely on data for many other things, including understanding or knowing how long we should stick something out. When you're frustrated with your boss in a meeting, you don't just get up and quit your job.

You can't walk away every time you get aggravated, irritated, or frustrated. Data teaches us that. But in other aspects of life, when there is a much larger "stay or leave" issue facing us down, we need to tap into all that we have learned up to this point to make that decision. We have to give ourselves the freedom to trust our spider senses, quiet our stakeholders, practice good gatekeeping, question the fables of our youths, and face our fears. That's how we think clearly about what we need to do. You will know how long to stick something out, in your gut, but more often than not, you will endure it for too long. By reflecting on what we have done, how we feel now, and what we want our lives to look like, we can use our data to inform our spider senses. Data will help you to learn how to sketch out what you want your life to look like, and to then determine the gap between where you are now and what you want in the future. Whether this is a new body, a new love, or a new life, these principles can help you get there.

WHAT IS DATA AND HOW DOES IT INFLUENCE YOU?

Simply put, data is information. So, a website, advice from your mom, and observing a coworker are all forms of data. Sometimes we actively search for data, and sometimes we encounter it by accident, or through someone else. It could be a billboard encouraging you to get a mammogram. The fact is, not all data has the same effect. Some data is objective or impersonal, such as a book or a website that gives you step-by-step advice. You won't feel as though you betrayed the book if you did or did not move forward with a decision. As such, that data does not damage your spider senses. In contrast, your mother may also strongly influence you. Data from her is different; it's less likely to be objective information, and much more likely to impact your spider senses.

As a scientist, I know we are not above emotion, even though the scientific method is meant to keep it honest. Even (and perhaps especially) in science, we may be invested in certain outcomes; we may even try to spin the data we collect in order to support findings that we want, even when the hard numbers don't support it. In fact, the way we protect against this in the scientific world is something we call peer review. Other people read our science and bring their own objectivity to bear, keeping us honest. In real life we don't have objective peer reviewers, but we do have lots of nonobjective folks that would love to weigh in.

Data is good. Nobel laureate and psychologist Daniel Kahneman's research, as well as the work of Harvard psychologist Daniel Gilbert, shows that we do well by sometimes getting other opinions. There are certain kinds of decisions we are not always equipped at making on our own. Our problem is that we don't always know how to consume that data. The trick is balance—balancing the data from the outside with what our spider senses dictate is best for us.

Let me use a dieting example. We receive a lot of data about food—nutrition wonks tell us what we should and should not eat, we learn about white carbs, bad fats, good oils, and on and on, until we are overwhelmed with the number of people telling us what we can and can't eat without knowing our preferences. This information comes at us from a world that tells us to look a certain way (which is another source of data). Then we need to balance this with our spider senses—when are we hungry, when are we full, what do we like to eat. It's a lot to balance. In the United States, people tend to eat in one of two ways. We either cut out everything forbidden—no sugar, no bread, no pasta, no dessert—or we just eat like drunken sailors, ordering everything and eating it without thinking about it. We lick our overfull plates clean. Many people find that they can't regulate themselves in the presence of challenging foods so they cut them out completely. Neither is a good idea. This entire book is about learning how to listen to yourself on the inside so you can handle the data that comes at you from the outside. You cannot control the toxic food world in which we reside, but you can control your response.

> *This entire book is about learning how to listen to yourself on the inside so you can handle the world that comes at you from the outside. You cannot control the toxic food world in which we reside, but you can control your response.*

LEARNING FROM EXPERIENCE

As we journey through life we accumulate data in the form of experiences. We learn what works and what doesn't. The wisest people use this experience and then reflect upon it to inform future decisions, but many of us just blindly hold on to the teachings of the past, despite what our experiences tell us. Confucius wisely says, "By three methods we may learn wisdom: First, by reflection, which is noblest; second, by imitation, which is easiest; and third by experience, which is the bitterest." Because imitation makes it easy to just do what we are taught, we find ourselves making the same mistakes again and again and not integrating the sometimes-bitter lessons of experience into the noble challenge of reflection.

DATA AND YOUR SPIDER SENSES

Sometimes gathering data and your spider senses may require taking the long view and making some tough choices. Even spider senses can pull you in different directions. This is where you need to occasionally face down some tough choices and ultimately learn from them so that you can make informed decisions in the future.

Jeff and Mary wanted to purchase a home in an expensive housing market and looked long and hard for a property. They resided in a small apartment in an urban neighborhood they loved, but they wanted to own their own house. They wound up getting frustrated, so Jeff suggested they start looking in outlying suburban areas. Mary wasn't convinced—her spider senses told her that moving away from friends and family was not a good idea—but she also wanted to do right by her husband. Her spider senses were all over the map. She felt like she was damned if she did and damned if she didn't; if she fought for what she felt was right and stayed in the city, even in a small place, she was afraid her husband would resent her. If she gave in and they moved, then she knew she wouldn't enjoy living in this new place, even if they had a lovely home. It was a catch-22. Mary was a pleaser and ultimately went along with the move to the suburbs. She hated it, felt isolated, and it caused tension between them. They eventually took the hit and sold the place. She felt that she had given it a chance; in essence, she collected data. It was a tough lesson, but ultimately a good one because Mary realized that her spider senses were dead-on all along, and she was also glad that she gave it a chance. It made her better able to trust herself down the road and she felt even more confident in her spider senses. It could be argued that she engaged in poor gatekeeping by choosing to live someplace she did not want, but I viewed it as a chance to use data and experience to inform future decisions. Past gatekeeping mistakes could be our best source of data, if we can just learn from them.

Sometimes our spider senses place us at an impasse. If we are lucky we get a chance to test out options. This may come at a cost; in Mary's case, this meant years of living away from family members and familiar places. But it also allowed her to give the option that mattered to Jeff a chance (which was also in line with her spider senses).

HOW TO USE DATA EFFECTIVELY

There are a couple of ways to use data. Some of us are data bingers: We ask everyone and their brother for advice, buy every book (I genuinely hope this will be the last advice book you'll ever need!), and traverse every website, and by the time we finish we are numb.

On the other hand, some of us are data dieters. We are afraid of data or feedback, so we don't seek any, and just move forward without taking the invaluable lessons of life and others with us.

The data dieters might be able to find success in their work if they are really listening to their spider senses. The fact is, if their spider senses are working, ideally they will be able to access and use data to act optimally while still honoring themselves. The fear of information overload can lead data dieters to miss some important and useful information. If your spider senses are on, then you can digest the data without losing yourself. The ideal balance involves making all decisions, particularly big-ticket, spider-sense-driven decisions yourself, by integrating data from your own past and from the outside in order to make a more prudent decision.

Let me give you an example. You may go ahead and quit your job to go back to culinary school based on what you know about yourself, but a little advice may help you score a better-suited program, or more financial aid. So, you understand the dream, but you pursue it more efficiently.

Here are the steps:

1.   Identify and state the problem.

2.   Generate a hypothesis on the basis of other people's data. This is basically what you think will happen.

3.   Collect the data.

4.   Draw some conclusions.

When we apply the scientific method to life, we need to tweak it a little bit.

1.   Identify the problem.

2.   Think about what you expect and what you are afraid of and then learn by watching others.

3.   Collect the data by not only listening to yourself, but, when necessary or prudent, by asking others and seeking out other sources of information as well. At this point it is important that you weigh these outside data, especially if they come from stakeholders, against what you know is right for you.

4.   Execute your plan.

Now let's see how you can apply this method to weight loss:

Step 1: I need to lose forty pounds. (Note: You've identified the problem.)

Step 2: I can't do it because I have never succeeded before. I love eating, I'm too busy, the kids make it difficult, and I hate to exercise. I will fail. The only thing I can do is starve myself and then I will lose weight. (Note: These beliefs are dangerous because they may trip you up, but if you listen to them, you may also learn more about your vulnerable areas and then pointedly address them.) For example, have the kids clear their plates so you don't eat their leftovers, and wake up fifteen minutes earlier in the morning to pack your lunch, so you don't buy calorie-rich foods at work.

Step 3: Make a food diary. Figure out your tough times of day. Speak to a dietitian. Find an exercise plan that you enjoy. Watch the eating habits and patterns of folks who have succeeded at maintaining a healthy weight. (Note: This is data.)

Step 4: On day one, toss out the junk food. On day two, start a food diary. On day three, drink two liters of water. (Note: You're executing your plan, solving your problem.)

You know you want to lose weight, and you know you have some hurdles to face, so you're going to use that data to develop a plan, evaluating the times of day you'll hit rough patches. You'll write down your foods in a log, collecting the data as you work toward achieving your goal or solving your problem. Then, with that data, you'll execute your plan, solving one problem a day, working toward the goal.

DATA AND DESSERT

Losing weight benefits tremendously from data, because it is a way of seeing change as well as tracking what trips you up. Food diaries are great because they not only reveal what you eat but also when you eat it. Willpower research tells us that you are more likely to start making mistakes later in the day, so food diaries show us when to kick up the mindfulness. They enable you to log changes—in your weight, in your dress size. They allow you to log times and situations that are challenging for you. They also help you to manage and organize your environment. If you know ice cream is your downfall, don't bring it into the house. If it's easy, you will eat it. I know that I have some places that still trip me up, and so when I can I avoid them, or I take the time to mentally prepare for them and talk my way through them if necessary.

There's a flip side to all this, which is where the spider senses come in. The scientific method we're using to collect the data to solve the problem is based in logic: Identify problems, use information, and draw conclusions. The problem is that most of our big-ticket decisions are not so logical, and, in fact, are generally muddied by emotion, which we have already established can impact our decision-making. Spider senses are not always logical. Selling all of your stuff and moving to Europe is not logical in light of long-term financial planning. Getting a divorce and raising kids alone with fewer financial resources is not logical. Ordering a steak and leaving two-thirds of it behind is not logical.

Here's the important part of this: Logic is not always right.

THE WHY

The trick to success is walking through the data minefield without blowing up, and to keep honoring your spider senses and integrating the data. Data can be your friend if you know how to use it properly. It can be your demise if you outsource your decisions to it and stop listening to yourself.

Spider senses and data are not incompatible; in fact, they benefit from each other. The data are the sails, and the spider senses are the wind. The spider senses push the boat to the destination, while the data guides you in how to make that change. But at the end of the day, the wind (spider senses) is what pushes the boat to its destination, while the data may prevent you from crashing on the rocks, allowing you to enter the harbor more smoothly and efficiently.

Be careful of stealth data. Marketers and the media are smarter than we are. We passively absorb the billboards, ads, and magazines that attack us at every turn. And with our smartphones and the Internet, we receive a steady diet of ads we aren't even consciously aware of: the wedding with the white dress, the granite countertops, the right car—just make sure they are what you want for you, and not what the world is telling you that you want.

Don't binge on data, and don't cut it out of your diet entirely. Just like with food, it's important to find that balance. Denial of data is often a way of not tackling the decision.

Remember, too, that data evolve, and while experience remains our greatest source of data, we have to remain open to other possibilities. The esteemed psychoanalyst Carl Jung once said, "Thoroughly unprepared, we take the step into the afternoon of life. Worse still, we take this step with the false presupposition that our truths and our ideals will serve us as hitherto . . . we cannot live the afternoon of life according to the program of life's morning, for what was great in the morning will be little at evening, and what in the morning was true, at evening will have become a lie." Basically, even in our own lives, that which once worked may not work in the future, or at any given point in time. Balance the data, but listen to yourself.

THE NOW

I want you to do an exercise in your journal, and it may take some time. This exercise will help to guide you through this book in a way that makes it most useful for you. Write down one big decision that is on your mind right now. Are you struggling with a relationship, or your weight, or maybe your career? Just think of something that really matters to you in your life.

In a separate place, write down what you want. Take a true moment to think about this one, quiet the voices, and just record what your spider senses say. For example, you may want to quit school. You are terrified, and that is reinforced by the fact that no one wants you to do it. It doesn't matter—just put that down if that's what you want. Be open about what you write down. Include anything related to your wants as well. Maybe you want to quit school because you hate your major, you don't want to live there, or you want to pursue your goals as a musician. Don't judge your reasons; there are enough other people doing that.

Now list all of the sources of data you could and typically would turn to for information on how to proceed. Here are some examples: family, friends, coworkers, the Internet (list specific websites if they would help in this process), spiritual advisor, health-care professionals, therapist, partner, mentor, children, guidebook, religious text, Reiki practitioner, book, song, television show—you name it.

Then list what you think they would advise you to do. Yes? Or Don't do it! Or You're crazy! Or Go for it! (You are likely to list different things next to different stakeholders and data sources.)

Now, rate the quality of advice you think they would give you on a scale of 1 to 10. A rating of 1 implies completely uninformed, naive advice, and 10 is expert wisdom.

Next, write down how you would feel if you did or did not listen to this data source. For example, you might feel guilty if you don't follow Mom's advice, and you might feel foolish if you don't heed the advice of a mentor. Connect the dots.

Think about which data sources will influence your spider senses—it doesn't mean you'll necessarily follow or ignore them, but you'll listen to them with a trained ear. Knowing the power of that data (advice from Mom can really influence you; advice from a book may not be as powerful), turn to the data that you think will be most useful. Tabulate it. Really assess your findings.

CHECK-IN: DATA

Here is some old-school decision-making work, but with a twist: the good old pros and cons list. These lists are simply a place to visually lay out the data you have acquired so you can make a decision. Take that thing you want to do and list out the pros and cons. Let's stick with the quitting-school example here.

Pros:

- You hate your program of study.

- It's too expensive.

- You want to pursue another goal.

Cons:

- You're concerned that not having a degree will hold you back.

- You really like your classmates.

Here's the new part: Your pros and cons list gets a third column, today and forevermore. It's the Spider Senses column. Make a note describing in detail what your spider senses tell you, because this means you have given the data its due, put it down, and thought about it. You have used it to inform what you may have known all along but perhaps now know in a more-informed way.

- This is not the school for me.

- I want to be a chef.

- I've always loved cooking.

As you read through this book, reflect back on this new style of pros and cons list, especially as you complete the remainder of the exercises. This book is one more source of data, so use it well to bolster your spider senses to achieve the body and life that you want.

CHAPTER 7

The Promise of One

Great things are not done by impulse, but by a series of small things brought together.

—Vincent van Gogh

"There's no way," she said. "I love food too much, I don't know how to say no, I hate the gym. I don't even know where to begin." I have heard these words, or some approximation of them, countless times from clients, acquaintances, even strangers on buses and airplanes. Many times clients come to me as the last stop on a long train ride involving dietitians, trainers, fad diets, juice machines, surgery, and medication.

Making change is overwhelming, and nowhere is this more pronounced than in the realm of weight loss and management. When you wake up one morning and decide to take on a seventy-five-pound weight loss, it seems impossible. You can't get your head around months of giving up sweets and going to the gym, but in fact, it is the sheer impossibility of getting your head around changing your life. And now we know that what seem like "small choices"—for example, saying no to dessert—are actually a dance through a minefield of the voices of others, fears from the past, present, and future, and the myths and scripts of our lives. So, what to do?

In the rest of this book, we are going to take the concepts of spider senses and gatekeeping and apply them to food, love, work, and life. But this isn't just about knowing—this is about doing. You know what you need to do; now I want you to do it. Use this book as a bridge to the life you want. I will start with a simple tool that will guide you through the journey we are about to take: the Promise of One.

It's simple. Does your life look the way you want it to look? No? Then enact your dreams with the Promise of One. It will show you how to take all that you will learn from reading this book and all of your experiences and make them work for you. I want your dreams to come true and your aspirations to be attempted. I want you to live the life you want to live, dance to your music, write your own script, listen to your body and feed it accordingly. Now that you are listening to your spider senses, the Promise of One will help you achieve the life you want. It will help you to overcome your fears, deal with your stakeholders, and knock out those infernal golden rules. It will help you to regain control and make you a better gatekeeper.

The Promise of One is based on goal-setting and goal-getting, and is actionable and powerful. It is my simple method of setting and accomplishing goals in all aspects of your life: food, job, money, dreams, and love. Instead of goal-setting, I like to think of it as dream-setting. Goals often feel sort of dull, but dreams feel powerful. Action can sometimes feel impossible, but the Promise of One guarantees that you will reach your goals and experience your dreams, not just think about them.

Goal-setting is at the core of motivation and regulating ourselves. Here is the prevailing wisdom on goals: You need to set two kinds of goals: short- and long-term. Each feeds on the other. If you are good at something, then set that goal high, but if it is new or you are not good at it, set the bar at a more-manageable level. If goals are set too high, the odds of failure, loss of self-esteem, and distress can stop us from reaching them. If they are set too low, we won't be motivated and they won't be gratifying. To wake up and say "I'm going to lose fifty pounds" is a lofty and overwhelming goal. That fifty-pound loss requires a series of daily goals, like eating more fruits and vegetables, watching portion size, moving every day, and hydrating. But daily goals can feel tedious, and long-term goals too far away.

We often feel "stuck"—so overwhelmed by the number of things that we want to change that we end up changing nothing. It's not possible to build a house in a day, but when you watch a building go up in your neighborhood, you see the daily progress. Weight loss and life are no different. By keeping this to one action per day, initially, it keeps the goal manageable and starts a new habit on its way. The Promise of One is about setting a foundation first—and this foundation is about taking the time and doing one thing each day.

What slowly happens is that the requirement starts becoming a part of your daily routine, and in fact, you may want to do more than one thing per day to get to where you want. You want to write a book or a screenplay? On the first day you may just write down a paragraph. And while it seems like it may take forever at that pace, as you take the time and start the process flowing—listening to yourself and slowly moving forward—you will find that one day, you can't stop yourself—the flow carries you forward much like a sailor catches the wind, and off you go. It means doing one thing every day—the size of the action is not important; it's the mindful and purposeful moment you take each day to bring about a change. It's a tribute to you. And ultimately, it is about momentum.

Action can sometimes feel impossible, but the Promise of One guarantees that you will reach your goals and experience your dreams, not just think about them.

THE WHY

The Promise of One is like planting a garden. Initially the process is slow; you till the soil, put down the seeds, dutifully water, and watch. Every day. In the beginning it can feel pointless—just taking care of dirt. Then one day the garden starts to flourish, flowers and fruits, blossoms and broccoli, and you can't keep up with all of it. You keep doing your part, and it starts paying off. The wonder of the Promise of One is that it stops feeling effortful, and before you know it, you grab the apple instead of the cookie. You exercise instead of sitting in front of the TV. You pursue goals instead of complaining about lost opportunities. And then one day, your new garden is actually a life full of new healthy habits. You are spending time in a way that moves you forward and in the direction of what you want for you, rather than avoiding life because you are afraid of taking on dreams and challenges.

At age thirty-nine, I set out to lose weight. For 510 days I did one thing a day, and over time, more. For example, one day I took the clothes off of the treadmill. The next day I walked five minutes on it. The day after that, I took the three flights of stairs to my office instead of the elevator for the short trip. The next day, I switched from soda to tea; the next, I bought a case of water. After that, I drank two liters a day. So as you can see, these are little things, but they added up to big change. Over time, doing one thing each day and listening to my spider senses turned these things into habits and also let me tweak the things that didn't feel right. Now I drink lots of water, but I'm not perfect and still succumb to the diet soda most days. Now I exercise nearly every day and always take the stairs, but I still struggle with food choices. The Promise of One helped me to shed eighty-five pounds and gain a new healthy body and life. Every day since, these once-a-day changes have developed into permanent habits. I still have moments when I struggle, but I have maintained my healthy weight for five years so far.

Two years ago, I reflected on my life, my patients, and my message, and decided that I wanted to write a book. Many people said no to me. For 365 days I did one of the following actions per day: e-mailing, researching, reading, writing, making phone calls, finding an agent. Then a publisher bought the book. The Promise of One turned into a dream— and the very book you hold in your hand.

THE NOW

The Promise of One is a daily method to break down your goals in a manageable way. Follow these steps:

Choose a dream and write it down. It can be something big like a fifty-pound weight loss, a vacation, producing a documentary, or running for mayor. Or it can be smaller, like losing ten pounds or cleaning out the garage.

Each day accomplish one thing toward that goal. This can be small some days, like eliminating all of the cookies and sweets from the house; searching the Internet to find out how much a plane ticket costs to your destination; or sending an e-mail about the evening photography classes at your local college. It's just one task per day, and it may only take two minutes. Log your steps in your smartphone, computer, or journal. For example:

Monday—tossed the sweets

Tuesday—bought strawberries

Wednesday—brought my healthy lunch to work

Thursday—walked four miles

Or it can look like:

Monday—e-mailed college

Tuesday—got response and returned e-mail

Wednesday—purchased book on photography

Thursday—read one chapter of book

Let the Promise of One guide you through the exercises at the end of each chapter as well. Even if you simply achieve one thing each day toward your dream, I promise you will make some significant shifts before you know it. Most important, you will find that taking these small steps toward your goal will become automatic, along with taking the time each day to step out of the mindless routine and turning it into mindful movement toward what you want for your life. Always listen to yourself—not just your spider senses, but anything that "interferes" with your spider senses or enacting your Promise of One. Perhaps you are afraid of failing (or succeeding), or your stakeholders are not supporting a change, or you are having trouble defying a long-held script like "Good students don't take a year off to travel." The beauty of the Promise of One is that you can often fight these big spider-sense scramblers by making smaller changes. On a day when you feel afraid of failing, make your "one thing" that you do more manageable. You are welcome to do more than one thing per day, but try to at least complete one step each day at a minimum. Label your journal accordingly: Day One, Day Two, and so on. You will be amazed at your progress over time.

CHECK-IN: PROMISE OF ONE

This is a simple check-in for you: *Just do it*. Build the Promise of One into your life. Take one new step a day to put you on the path toward your goal. Ideally, I'd suggest you do it in the morning, because one step might lead to more steps that day, like a response from a job inquiry, for example. If you download the app that goes along with this book, you'll have the option of having me nudge you once a day, reminding you to do that one thing and get to the life you want. No excuses. After each chapter, think about the takeaway message of that chapter and use the Promise of One to enact it in a manageable way. One day you throw out the sweets, another day you eat half the sandwich, another day you buy smaller bowls, and so forth.

PART TWO:
Join the Dirty-Plate Club

CHAPTER 8

How Do You Eat?

I cannot remember the books I've read any more than the
meals I have eaten; even so, they have made me.

—Ralph Waldo Emerson

You think you're reading this because you want to lose weight, and I am
confident you will, largely by learning to walk away and leaning on your
spider senses rather than your fears, the golden rules, and your stakeholders when making decisions about eating. But I promise you that once we
lift up the hood and see what's underneath, you're going to learn about
some other important elements in your life, including:

- relationships,

- work, and

- how you spend your money.

My hope is that as you read this book, you'll reap the same benefits
my patients do when they walk into my office and learn to use these
techniques. Even though reading a book is not the same as sitting across
from each other, the self-realization and transformation will be just as
powerful.

Let's take a look at the basics to determine exactly what kind of eater
you are and the influences you have confronted in your life with regard
to food. Let's understand you. And be honest. This is the self-assessment

stage. To really understand yourself and your eating, don't write down how you *want* to eat; write down how you actually do eat. Once we understand this, we'll fix it by the end of this book, I promise. This chapter involves doing the exercises as you read through it. I would recommend reading it once and taking it all in, and then circling back and rereading it with your journal by your side, so you can complete the exercises.

WHO, WHAT, WHEN, WHERE, WHY, AND HOW DO YOU FILL YOUR PLATE?

Let me ask you some questions and help you start this journey to a place where you can trust the finely honed machine that is you, and create life as you want it, instead of the life others want for you.

It all starts with what you put on your plate and how you eat it.

Who?

The fundamental question here is: How do other people influence how you eat? Remember, the people who influence you are your stakeholders.

People are food cues. Take a moment and reflect on how your eating habits differ depending on your company. Some people want you to eat the way they eat. Others don't care. In addition, people can influence the decisions you make about food: the mother who asks you why you aren't eating more, the aunt who tells you to eat less, the father who still wants you to clean your plate, or the girlfriend who chastises you for not ordering dessert. Their words and wishes can lead you to ignore your wants, your knowing, and your spider senses.

MY EATING HABITS

Now get out your journal and answer a few questions. You can answer: never, sometimes, most of the time, or all of the time.

- How often do you eat alone?
- How often do you eat with others?
- How often do you eat with children under the age of twelve?

Now let's do some comparisons, and here I want you to think about how you typically eat—*typically* meaning an average meal, the majority of the time.

- When you eat alone, how well do you eat? (Worse than usual, the same as usual, better than usual)

- When you eat with other people, how well do you eat? (Worse than usual, the same as usual, better than usual)

- When you eat with children, how well do you eat? (Worse than usual, the same as usual, better than usual)

Now, let's think about the people you eat with. Some of them are what I term "gut-busters"—the people who can throw off your spider senses with their words, their own eating habits, or even your history with them. List some of those people now—the people who make it hard for you to really honor yourself at the table—and when you list them, think about some of the reasons why that happens.

For example, your answers might look like this:

> Gut-buster: Mary from the office
> Why: She always orders appetizers and an entree and dessert, and she gives me a hard time when I don't do the same.
> Result: I find myself ordering more than I intended and feeling guilty during and after the meal.

Now list your spider-sense supporters—the people who lead you to eat better, or, at the very least, the people with whom you do not feel compelled to eat in any way except the way you want. Here's an example:

> Supporter: My pal Lori
> Why: She doesn't really care. I eat with her to enjoy her company and she enjoys mine. We talk more than we eat during the meal, and she rarely wants dessert.
> Result: We often share an entree. I feel silly having dessert when she doesn't, and I leave these meals feeling full from the conversation instead of the food.

MISTAKE METER

Which people do you find you most often make decisions with? I want you to really reflect on these answers in the Who category.

- Are there major (or even minor) differences in your patterns of eating, filling your plate, and what you eat depending on who you are eating with?

- Do children (yours or someone else's) influence your eating?

- Do you take on the eating habits of those around you—and if so, whose habits do you take on—or are you consistent?

Take a moment and reflect on how your spider senses are affected by whom you eat with, and who most throws off your spider senses when you are eating. These are the people with whom you may need to take a moment and let your spider senses breathe, so you can learn to eat with them while still listening to yourself.

Review your answers so you can think about making some changes. If you are aware that you will be seeing a gut-buster, prepare yourself mentally ahead of time so you can be steadfast with a dining companion that tends to overeat. If you are going to a restaurant with a person who usually over-orders, or takes over ordering for everyone, go online and look at the menu ahead of time so you can cut that person off at the pass and ensure that there are some healthy options at the table.

If you find yourself struggling with kids and their food (many parents idly eat lots of calories off of their children's plates of macaroni and cheese), first take a step back and strive to make sure there are healthy options for your children. Also, you want to welcome your kids into the dirty-plate club, so model it for them. If they have eaten well and are done, don't be shy about throwing away what's left on their half-full plates (instead of eating off of them). Ideally, you teach your children good gatekeeping—when possible to order a smaller portion or serve themselves a smaller portion. If that is not possible, do not turn yourself into a trash receptable for what they did not finish. It results in two mistakes: down the road they may feel compelled to finish everything because they have seen you do it, and in the short-term, those extra calories often get forgotten, but your body doesn't know they aren't coming off of your own plate.

If you are feeling stressed, depleted, or fatigued but want to go out with a friend for a meal, reflect on your journal answers, and select a friend who is not a gut-puncher, but instead an easy eater, or even a non-eater. Sometimes a meal is the price of sharing a conversation. We rarely say "Let's get together to talk"—we usually go out for lunch, dinner, coffee, or drinks. Obviously sharing meals is wonderful, but sometimes our bodies and minds just need companionship. Interestingly, I have a friend who is struggling with her weight. Recently she said, "I want to see you but I don't want to sit down and eat, which seems to be the only reason people get together." She asked me if I would be willing to get together to take walks. Now we get together and have the same (if not better and richer) conversations, without finding ourselves eating and drinking as a way of getting together. Try to find other innovative ways (e.g. movies without popcorn, museums), especially with your gut-punchers, to keep the social contact going without having the calories flowing.

What?

Calories are calories. Period. We lose weight by burning more calories than we consume. We know that a pound of lettuce contains fewer calories than a pound of chocolate or a pound of steak, but this is not meant to be a nutritional analysis. What we eat has to do with issues such as personal preferences, health, availability, and cost, as well as subtle emotional issues, including what makes us feel good, what comforts us, numbs us, and reminds us of something good or someone who took care of us.

Some foods are efficient: They are full of nutrients and they satiate us, therefore carrying us for a longer period of time. Some foods simply fill us up sooner. Some burn down fast. But what we eat usually has more to do with what we feel about it than some elegant nutritional decision-making.

This next exercise is sort of fun. Take a minute and (a) list your *favorite* foods in your journal. Don't think about it—just list them. Nobody is reading your journal but you, and this self-assessment is about being honest. Don't write down broccoli and skinless chicken. I'll get you started and fess up to mine now: Neapolitan pizza, lasagna, cheesecake, chili, all Indian food, dim sum, and cheeseburgers. Love them all.

Now (b) write down what you typically eat. What are your daily go-to foods. They'll vary, we know that, but in general, I suspect your breakfasts are often the same and maybe even your lunches. We are creatures of habit.

Next, write down what you think you're (c) supposed to eat based on all you've heard from the pundits, the nutrition segments on TV, the magazines, and all the good-food-up-in-your-facers who preach what you should eat. In other words, if you were being good, what does an aspirational food day look like to you?

Finally, (d) list any foods that make you feel out of control, that when you see them you can't stop eating them—when just a little isn't an option.

Write down your favorite meal. What is it? What feelings does this meal evoke for you? Why is it your favorite? How often do you have it? Who does it remind you of? Where do you typically eat it? When you eat this meal, how are your spider senses working? Is this a meal that helps you be better able to honor your sense of being full? Does it help you make good choices?

On a scale of 1 to 10 (1 being never, 10 being all the time), write down what proportion of the time you eat the foods you want to eat.

How do you feel when you eat the foods that you want to eat? Some feelings may include:

- Soothed

- Anxious

- Out of control

- In control

- Guilty

- Happy

- Angry

- Bored

- Satisfied

- What else?

Really consider this question: How do you feel when you can't eat the foods that you want to eat? Do you feel:

- Frustrated

- Bitter

- Happy

- Angry

- Indifferent

- Deprived

- In control

- Out of control

- Virtuous

- What else?

MISTAKE METER

What foods are you the most out-of-control with? Eating is a two-way street: It drives and is driven by our emotions. In theory, everyone can eat anything he or she wants—it's about quantity. If you want steak, eat a four-ounce portion; it looks a bit lonely on the plate, but you can have it. Deprivation leads us to behave badly, and some foods make us feel out-of-control. Reflect on what you think you are supposed to eat, what you do eat, what you want to eat, what you like to eat, and how well your spider senses work with these various foods.

As for those foods that are the hardest for you, don't kick them out of your life, but don't move them in either. Try not to keep them in the house, but allow them from time to time. When you go to a restaurant, order what you want, but learn how to either ask for less or throw half of it away. When you only allow yourself the foods you are supposed to eat—which may not always be the foods you find most palatable—then over time, when you finally encounter your beloved foods, you will feel out-of-control and perhaps even a bit scared that you won't see them again for a long time, so you may overeat. Create a balance. Bring in the foods you love and balance them with options that really round things out nutritionally. For example, have that slice of fabulous pizza with a big salad. Really relish the pizza, eating it slowly and making it last, and then let the salad complement the meal.

When?

Different times of day yield different eating patterns. The classic pattern is what I call the aspirational morning followed by the dark night of the soul. By that I mean you wake up ready to take on your healthy eating edicts: egg whites, fruit, lean dairy, and whole wheat. Every day is a fresh start. However, not every day goes the way you want. Sometimes you are so busy in the morning that you may skip breakfast altogether, and in the midst of trying to get through your morning, don't feel hungry or deprived. The day goes on, stress kicks in, more meals may get skipped, but you are hungry and foods that you didn't choose may be offered by others (donuts in the coffee room). You start to eat to avoid the struggles of the day, and by nighttime you may eat because you are frustrated, bored, lonely, or just hungry from not eating all day. Most people make more food mistakes as the day progresses. We will discuss why that happens shortly. It varies from person to person, and it's important to figure out what times of day most affect you.

WHEN I EAT

How often do you eat breakfast (number of mornings per week)? How often do you eat dinner, dessert, or a snack after 9 p.m. (number of nights per week)? Try to make a little chart to determine the percentage of calories that you eat in a day at various times. For example:

Breakfast—zero

Lunch—15 percent

Afternoon snack—35 percent

Dinner—20 percent

Evening snack (after 9 p.m.)—30 percent

Your eating day should strive to look more like this:

Breakfast—30 percent (between 6 and 10 a.m.)

Lunch—35 percent (between 11:30 a.m. and 2:30 p.m.)

Afternoon snack—10 percent (between 2:45 and 4:45 p.m.)

Dinner—25 percent (between 6 and 9 p.m.)

Rank the quality of your eating from 1 to 10 at each time of day (1 being really bad, out-of-control, or unhealthy, and 10 being healthy, balanced, and controlled). Also, keep in mind that your weekend eating will look a bit different than your weekday eating.

MISTAKE METER

Using your journal, reflect on what time of day you make the worst food decisions. Timing, as they say, is everything, so really take the time to reflect upon the differences in your patterns of eating, filling your plate, and how you eat depending on the time of day, and even the time of year. Seasonally, you should note if you eat more during the holidays, during the winter months, or on weekends. Also, are there times of the day when you find it easier to walk away from your plate when you are full, and are there times when you just can't stop yourself?

Now that you know your more-challenging eating times and you've taken a look at your rhythms, it's time to reflect on when your spider senses are the most off. (You will probably notice that it is when you're making the poorest food decisions.) It may also be a time of day when you have more stakeholders around (e.g., dinner), or you tend to be more impacted by fear (e.g., end-of-day stress and anxiety). If you eat badly when you're home at night, reconfigure your environment and try to get the more-challenging foods out of the house. If you skip breakfast but then overindulge at the coffee cart at work, then wake up earlier and try to give yourself better choices at home. When you know your tricky times, you can practice better mindfulness then. This is about being aware of the *when* so you don't blindly make bad choices at challenging times.

Where?

Simply put: We eat everywhere. We eat in the living room, in our beds, in our cars, walking, talking, at our desks, in restaurants, standing in front of an open fridge, at the counter, on the beach—you name it. The problem: That's not a good thing. We need to show some control in order to be more mindful. Imagine if you could just feed your urge to have sex anywhere. (Well, maybe you do, but that's for another book.) Seriously, we restrain ourselves with other urges, but rarely with food. We regulate our appetites for other things and restrict them to certain settings, but we have a lot of trouble doing that with food.

Let's take a page out of how we help people who have trouble falling asleep. The first thing we do is engage in something called *stimulus control*. That means making the bed solely a place for sleeping. Many of us do everything in our beds—watch TV, surf the Internet, read, eat—and as such, the bed can become a confused space. Thus, to address this we take everything else out of that space, clean it up, dim the lights, and make our bed about sleep. It's a similar thing with food, so I try to find out from clients where they eat badly.

To understand your where habits, reflect on the following using a scale of 1 to 10 (where 1 is never and 10 is all the time). Make notes in your journal:

- How often do you eat at home?
- How often do you eat outside the home?
- When you eat outside the home, how often do you bring your own food?
- How often do you dine in restaurants?
- How often do you eat in your car or while walking?

Think about how you typically eat. *Typically* means an average meal, the majority of the time. That is your usual meal.

- When you eat at home, how well do you eat? (Worse than usual, the same as usual, better than usual)
- When you eat while "on the go" (e.g., walking around, in your car), how well do you eat? (Worse than usual, the same as usual, better than usual)
- When you eat out, how well do you eat? (Worse than usual, the same as usual, better than usual)

Now within your home or office, really consider the following places and how often you eat in these places:

- Kitchen table / bar counter
- Standing up or over the sink
- Some other dining table
- Living room couch
- Desk
- Bed
- Bedroom
- Patio or outdoor area
- Other location in home/office
- Where else?

MISTAKE METER

In what places do you have the most difficulty regulating your eating? Where do you eat worse than usual? More than you intended? Not all places are created equal, and some of us have more trouble in some places than others. Spider senses are again kind of like your cell phone. There are places where it works and places where it doesn't. Places we eat are similar, in that some mess with our spider senses. In general, try to stick to eating at eating places, like the kitchen table. When you look at your ratings and patterns, I think you'll notice that you tend to make better food decisions and eat more reasonably there.

We also sometimes neglect to count the calories we eat at spots other than eating places. Reflect also on the types of mistakes you make while eating out versus eating at home. Remember that when you eat out, you have less say about what ends up on your plate, and this can lead you to eat more than you intended. If you are headed to a "bad food location" (e.g., your car, your office), you may want to eat something healthy at home before you get there, so you'll be less likely to succumb to your usual patterns in those places. Keep the food out of those places: Take the chips out of the car, the chocolates out of your desk. Mindless eating takes place in these locations, and by taking away the stimulus, you will be better able to avoid eating in those locales. If you find that you eat badly in certain kinds of restaurants, watch how you order. Be mindful and slow down. Go ahead and get that favorite dish, but complement it with steamed vegetables or greens or something that may fill you up and make the meal last longer.

Why?

It should be simple, right? You eat because you're hungry. Not so much, though. In fact, I'm guessing that you eat because you are hungry less than 50 percent of the time. Grab your journal again and let's write down the why's of your eating. Some reasons, instead of hunger, could be:

- Food still on the plate
- Food being offered (e.g. grocery store samples, food being passed at a party)
- It's time to eat according to the clock, your boss, or others
- Reward (you had a good presentation so you deserve a treat)
- Frustration

- Loneliness

- Anger

- Anxiety

- Boredom

- Happiness

- Depression

- Stress

- Comfort

- You want to try a new food

- Other people's pressure to eat

You probably have other reasons as well. Now, of the reasons you listed, circle or check the ones that cause you to eat most often.

Now let's consider reasons you stop eating. Make a list, but use the following as examples:

- You're full.

- Your plate is empty.

- Others stopped eating.

- You don't like the food.

- You're sticking to your portion-controlled diet.

- You're short on time and can't finish.

- You feel sick.

- You've finished watching your show on TV.

- You've finished reading what you were reading.

- Your children interrupted or needed help with something.

- You took a phone call.

Again, you might have other reasons as well. Circle or check the reasons that most often stop your consumption. But the big question here is how often are you able to stop eating and perhaps leave food on your plate when you're full? And if you don't eat it all, how often are you willing to leave behind the leftovers? I want you to really think about that.

MISTAKE METER

What are your three non-hunger reasons for ignoring your spider senses, and what is the main reason you don't stop eating when you're done? If you can understand all the non-hunger-driven reasons that you eat, then you can start targeting those reasons. Also, when you're not eating for nourishment, you're often eating for other psychological reasons, and that's when we really go for the bad stuff like sugars, fats, comfort foods, and fried snacks. Whenever I want to eat something, I enact something I call the "apple test." I reflect on whether fruits, vegetables, or a healthy option would work. If I truly need to eat out of hunger, those options would be just fine, and I would welcome them. If I am eating for other reasons, I tend to gravitate to the junk. At that point I'm not eating for reasons related to food; I'm eating for some other psychological reason that is not meant to be addressed by food.

Once you figure out the non-hunger reasons for not eating, write them all down on a Post-it note and put those notes on the cabinets in the kitchen, on your computer at work, on the dashboard of your car—wherever you are when you make your food mistakes. This is a daily task that has to happen each and every time you reach for food. Ask yourself, Why am I choosing this? The fact is, if you can master your why, you have mastered this problem. You can find alternative ways to address these needs, and you can stop outsourcing your dreams to a piece of cake. This means listening to yourself. Most of us in our culture stopped listening to ourselves long ago, for all the reasons we have discussed—stakeholders, fears, and golden rules. If our thinking is not in line with all of that, then it's easier to stop thinking. This mindlessness is the core of most people's eating issues. Figure out the why, and you can take a new approach to gatekeeping, listening to your body, and enjoying food and life in a new way.

How?

Channel your inner Dr. Seuss here and assess the how of eating: with a fork, with a spoon; in a car or in your room; fast or slow or in between; at the table or on the go.

We've become so programmed to just shoveling it in wherever and whenever that we seem to take for granted how we eat. The how is one of the big reasons we don't often monitor our eating, and why we don't eat well. Do you ever order Chinese food, stand at the counter, and eat half the carton of fried rice, and then scoop another meal-size portion out and eat it at the table? You've just eaten twice. Do you eat at your desk most days for lunch and simply forget what you ate, because you did it so mindlessly while sending e-mails or doing paperwork quickly between meetings?

Let's rate how you eat. Use your journal to consider the following three choices:

When you're not eating for nourishment, you're often eating for other psychological reasons, and that's when we really go for the bad stuff, like sugars, fats, comfort foods, and fried snacks.

- Slowly and mindfully

- Average but distracted

- Rushed and mindlessly

Now, using these three choices, assess:

- What's the average pace of how you eat?

- How do you typically eat at home?

- How do you typically eat at a restaurant or in front of others?

The *how* of eating is linked in large part to the *where* and the *who*. Do you set the table when you eat alone at home, or do you take up residence on the couch? Does solitary mealtime lack ceremony? We don't often consider it worthwhile to set out plates and make a fuss over a quick meal, or dinner for one, but making it special can create mindful—instead of mindless—eating.

MISTAKE METER

What situations are associated with the most rushed, mindless eating for you? Think of places, times, people, and situations. Think about the patterns in how you eat. Do utensils slow you down? For example, sandwiches are tricky because grab-and-go foods tend to get consumed more quickly than food that requires cutting or spooning. Does it help to have the table set? What types of meals, foods, and settings lead you to eat more quickly, or slowly?

YOUR CHILDHOOD DINNER TABLE

The crux of our current eating patterns, the place where we learned all of our habits, is the childhood table. It's where the emotions associated with food really congealed for us all. It's where we learned to eat too much or too little. Some of us were taught that eating food meant love for the person serving or cooking it. Many of us learned it was (and is) imperative that we clean our plates. Some of us were made to feel badly about the way we ate or what we were eating. Others found food and the table to be a place of connection.

I spend a lot of time with clients trying to find out what a typical night at the childhood dinner table was like for them. Let's do that for you now by having you answer in your journal the following questions:

- Who was typically there?

- How often did you eat together?

- What was it like?

- What was served?

- What happened if you didn't finish what was on your plate?

- What did food mean when you were growing up?

- Who filled your plate?

- Where did you eat?

The lessons from the childhood dinner table often transcend food. They taught us about whether we were heard, how feelings were communicated, who the stakeholders were, the golden rules, our sense of power, and what was expected of us. And because it is a place where we honed very primitive senses about how full we were, these voices and lessons often carried over not only to the dinner tables we find ourselves at presently, but also into our bedrooms, offices, and homes.

Put away your diet books and the foods you hate. This time start by asking six simple questions about eating and food: Who, What, When, Where, Why, and How? This is about understanding the rhythms of your eating habits. They have become so ingrained and so habitual that until you really break it down, you will not become aware of your vulnerabilities. Most important, monitor how the Who, What, When, Where, Why, and How impact and are impacted by your spider senses. By figuring out when you are most vulnerable to making mistakes, you can ratchet up your mindfulness at those times. You may always get it right at the breakfast table at home, so relax there, but it is that damned drive-through window you hit after a long day that undoes you—that's when you need to pay attention.

As you go through the exercises in this chapter, keep in mind that no one will see your answers—this is about a private and honest space where you can address your patterns in a truthful manner.

YOUR FOOD MOMENT

Many people remember a moment when they started thinking differently about food, or their weight. For some people it was an insensitive comment from a parent; for others, teasing by friends. It could have come in adulthood from a spouse/partner, or from an adolescent child. It could have been an employer or an athletics coach. But there is that food "moment," and in my years of working with clients on food issues, I've found that they all remember their moment. This is when it turns, the script shifts, and your spider senses are thrown. The script can be shifted back, and the first step is to identify that moment and start reframing.

Ask yourself, What was the moment? What happened? How did it impact my food attitude and body image? How does it still affect how I relate to food and my body today? If you still have regular contact with the person (or situation), then you may be more likely to keep replaying that script in your head. Remain mindful of this and allow it to have less of a hold on your spider senses.

THE WHY

This not just about why, but it's about all the things that surround why you eat. By breaking it down you may find out that you do eat when you are hungry and are able to honor that spider sense, but the who is what throws you off. It's different for each of us.

THE NOW

This is where your new food journey begins. It's no longer about simply counting calories and eating what other people tell you to eat. For the first time you are going to listen to your body. You know more about you than anybody else. At the beginning of this chapter I reminded you to read it and take it in. Now go back, armed with all of this information, and really do it.

CHECK-IN: HOW DO YOU EAT

You already did the heavy lifting by doing all of the exercises in this chapter. The key is to use these answers as a framework every day. Each day, each time you have to make a food choice, do a quick assessment of the Who, What, Where, When, Why, and How. It takes less time than you think, and now that you have laid out the road map of your personal eating land mines, you are going to be better able to face down those situations and let your spider senses do their work. The next few chapters will give you the tools you need to work within the structure of your life, your settings, your people, and your schedule—no more eating in a way that suits others; it's time to listen to you.

CHAPTER 9

Brains, Behavior, and Bagels

The glory of science is, that it is freeing the soul, breaking the mental manacles, getting the brain out of bondage, giving courage to thought, filling the world with mercy, justice, and joy.

—Robert G. Ingersoll

Let's try to break our brains and bodies out of bondage. When it comes to weight loss, we may feel doomed to fail; it may even feel like a conspiracy. In this chapter, you will learn that your brain may be in on this conspiracy. This is a book about spider senses, about the fact that you are actually wired to do this. So let's take a quick look under the hood at your brain, behind the "science" of spider senses, of eating, and of why eating and walking away from anything can be such a tough nut to crack.

HABITS

Most adults gain one to two pounds per year between the ages of twenty and sixty years, as reported by Hill and colleagues in the journal *Science*. That means on average you can expect to be forty to sixty pounds heavier at sixty than you were at twenty just by doing the same thing over time. It will be harder to lose weight with each passing year. From my seat as a clinician, and as a woman, this has been my experience, both for my clients and me.

Spider senses make us efficient, and so do habits. Even if our eating habits don't change one bit, over time we are going to gain weight. We don't think about a lot of the daily stuff we do—we just do it. Habits can be healthy (teeth brushing) or unhealthy (smoking), but they are things we often do without thinking. When it comes to eating, what really gets us is that many of us are "trained" to look for food at certain times—lunch, midafternoon, and late at night. And that will often override our spider senses.

MOTIVATION

Motivation asks the simple question, "Why?" Why do we eat? There are many theories out there about motivation, but in basic terms, motivation helps activate, focus, and maintain our behavior. Some of our motivation is innate, meaning it is biological; some is incentive based, meaning it is driven by reward; and then there is what we call cognitive, which is how you and I interpret things that have happened. We know that there are some basic drives most people have—to be safe, to not feel hungry or thirsty, to be with other people, to achieve, to create, to rest, to please. These drives lead us to behave in certain ways. If we can understand what motivates us, then we can change it.

For each of us, what motivates us to do anything, including eating, varies. Some people work to make money to buy things. Some people work to impress others. Some people work because they love what they do. You can see how different drives or motivations to work will result in a different approach to work, different interpretations of events at work, and so on.

So let's think about food. In theory we should eat to nourish ourselves; that is the drive that food is designed to address. But as is clear, that's only a small reason many of us are motivated to eat. We use food as a tool for other things—for example, eating is often how we spend time with other people. Social affiliation is an important need, and food often becomes tangled up in the web of meeting another need.

Our motivations are dictated not only by the world outside of us but by the world inside of us as well. We have to learn to eat in a toxic food environment (outside of us) while having to manage our particular motivations and triggers (inside of us). Both of these issues represent a unique challenge, and the outside world is unlikely to change. So that leaves only the option of learning to respond differently to the outside world while learning about our specific weaknesses and triggers.

Outside world ⟶ **HOW WE EAT** ⟵ **Inside world**

At the end of the chapter, and this is something we have already done, we will again address why you eat. Motivational theories tell us that we eat for lots of reasons, and by using food as a tool for something it wasn't designed to do, we may end up consuming more of it. The bottom line, though, beyond hunger, is that one of the reasons we eat (and eat too much) is because it is rewarding. Let's talk about rewards.

THE REWARD

Our brains love pleasure. Dopamine is the pleasure neurotransmitter, and when we do something that feels good—food, drugs, sex—dopamine is what makes us want to do it again (and again). We aren't foolish; things that feel good get repeated, and our brains are in on this. We know that certain kinds of foods—sugary, fatty, salty—tend to have more of an impact on the reward centers in our brains. And that reward has a big lead-up to it. Just knowing that we are getting the cheesecake can get the dopamine firing. This means that once we actually face down the cheesecake, we tend to eat more of it. The brain is like a spoiled child and often gets what it wants.

What happens inside our brains translates into behavior. If we do something and get rewarded for it, we are going to do it again. If we eat a burger and it tastes good, we will eat another burger; if we eat our mother's cooking and she is so happy that it fills us with a warm, fuzzy feeling, we will eat more. This is called positive *reinforcement*. Many of us entered the world of eating with good intentions—we would eat because things tasted good and we were hungry. But over time, we learned some bad things about how to use food. Many people use food to avoid bad feelings. This is called negative *reinforcement*—we eat to take away a bad feeling, or, at the very least, to distract ourselves from it or to numb ourselves.

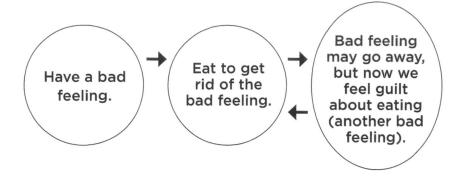

What's hard about eating is that it is kept in place by both positive and negative reinforcement. Here is where I want you to think about the rule of FLAB: The main reasons many of us eat are to deal with feelings of **F**rustration, **L**oneliness, **A**nxiety, and **B**oredom. Over time, when we have those feelings, we reflexively know that food will remove them, so we indulge in those comfort foods. (How many broken hearts have been treated by pints of ice cream?) Eating becomes a one-two punch. It makes us feel good and it takes away bad feelings. And as said earlier, this is how it can become a habit. When you have a bad day at work, you walk in the door, open a bag of chips, and you feel momentarily better.

It's rewarding to see the people around us happy, even if that means not listening to ourselves; it's also rewarding not to have to deal with unpleasant emotions, like fear. As such, the very things that damage our spider senses (e.g., stakeholders) are often what reward our eating. So by eating, we mute our spider senses and move further away from listening to ourselves. The rewarding aspects of food can lead us to eat in a patterned way, blindly and without thinking. And that can interfere with willpower and self-regulation.

The rewarding aspects of food can lead us to eat in a patterned way, blindly and without thinking. And that can interfere with willpower and self-regulation.

WHERE THERE'S A WILL THERE'S A WAY

Willpower, self-regulation, and self-control are all ways of saying *just do it* (or *don't do it,* as the case may be). Deprivation equals failure when it comes to weight management, and yet deprivation likely drives weight loss and management (and life) approaches for most people. Research on willpower shows that it's not that simple. Willpower is a finite resource, like gas in a tank, and it can get used up. When we are tapped out or depleted, we make bad decisions. On any given day we may wake up and eat egg whites and fruit, and later that day find ourselves mindlessly eating ice cream out of the carton.

What sorts of things deplete willpower? According to Baumeister, interestingly, willpower is what depletes willpower. The more we are forced to regulate ourselves, the harder it gets. A day spent regulating what we eat and what we say, and being disciplined about lots of other things leaves us feeling depleted. Keep in mind that self-regulation requires the brain to do its job, and guess what the fuel of the brain is? Glucose. Sugar. Experiments looking at willpower show that when you give a person some sugar, they are less likely to succumb to temptation when given the option. So paradoxically, if you want to be better equipped to make choices, keep yourself fed. We often feel virtuous when we deprive ourselves while in truth, deprivation often leads us to behave far less virtuously.

The stuff of life depletes us as well—deadlines, work, kids, friends, family, stress—and when we expend resources to keep it together in our lives, it's easier to succumb to bad food choices. I actually think the only reason that spa-based weight-loss programs work—when you check into a beautiful space, do yoga, and relax—is because the cares of your daily life are behind you, and someone else is preparing the menu. *Of course* you can tolerate healthy choices 24/7 when you have no other distractions or stressors. And subsequently, you lose weight. Then you get home, and in the midst of traffic jams, screaming stakeholders, and bills to pay, you start reaching for the bad stuff, and the weight returns. Then you deem yourself a failure. But that's not true; you are just back to your depleted self, and your ability to make healthy choices or exert willpower diminishes.

Lots of people who are trying to lose weight often fail when they "fall off the wagon." They declare a mandate: "No white sugar." They change nothing else about their lives—they have the same stressors, same problems. It's a recipe for failure. Then one day, they eat a piece of cake, and they say, "Well, I've failed—to hell with it, I'm going to just eat anything I want." And the cycle begins anew. Eating occurs in a context—of your world, of your life—and making healthy choices is not just about saying yes or no; it's about realizing that there are times when it's harder to regulate yourself, not just with food, but with everything.

In chapter 4, we talked about Baumeister's important work on willpower. Remember, willpower can also be tapped out by the very things that tap out our spider senses—fears, golden rules, and those stakeholders. Fears and stakeholders in particular can sometimes deplete us, making demands on us, and then we may be less able to control ourselves at times of weakness. Does this mean that all is lost? If willpower is in fact a limited resource, does that mean we're doomed? No.

We have a way to fight this, and it's simple. By knowing that willpower does get depleted and that it's not because we are "weak," but because our brains need energy and we need a break, we can be a little kinder to ourselves. What's the trick to beating back these lapses in willpower that throw us off?

Stop, Look, Listen . . . Then Eat

We like to flatter ourselves when we're busy, and think that we're multitasking. Actually, what we are doing is multi-failing. By paying attention to many things, we are paying attention to none. When we multitask, or simply don't pay attention, we go on autopilot and do certain things—like eating—mindlessly. Thus, when willpower is depleted, most of our other resources, including attention, are depleted too, so we end up not paying attention and succumbing to the "fix." This is probably the most challenging thing that this book will ask of you: to stop, look, and listen (to yourself) before you eat. It won't be easy to do, and it may seem silly at first, but if you practice it, over time it will become a habit. Here are some tips on how to stop before you eat:

- Never eat out of the package; go through the motions of putting an actual serving on a plate.

- Drink an 8- to 12-ounce glass of water before you eat; it slows you down and creates a sense of fullness. It can also jump start the mindfulness by allowing you to pause before you eat.

- If you have to keep forbidden foods in the house, put them up high or lock them up. That moment of having to pull a circus act to get them will slow you down.

- Use Post-its or other reminders around your kitchen, office, car, or wherever else you make food mistakes. Write down a question that makes you stop, look, and listen to your spider senses. (My Post-it says *Why are you doing this?*)

The Mindfulness Minute

It doesn't have to be a full minute—it could be thirty seconds. Right before you start eating, take three long, deep, slow breaths and pay attention to yourself. What are you feeling? Think about the rule of FLAB, and whether it could be any of those emotions. At the end of this chapter, I will ask you to make a list of distracter activities (that do not involve food); try one of those instead. Just taking that short moment can put your attention where it belongs, and even if you feel depleted and your willpower is low, this mindfulness minute can help you stop and think. By doing this, you could avoid hundreds of mindless calories per day.

So through the exercises in this chapter and by understanding the how of eating, you can start to identify those periods of the day when you need to pay attention. Be mindful. Wait a moment before eating or reaching. Create environments where it is less easy to mindlessly grab junk food. This is not just about being more "disciplined"; once again, as with your spider senses, it is about honoring yourself, and your rhythms.

AVOIDING INERTIA EATING

Mistakes don't happen all at once—there are steps in the process. The earlier in the process (gatekeeping) we can stop, the better our chances of beating them back. Let's take a look at a common mistake many of us make: late-night snacking and your probability of stopping yourself from overeating on the sofa.

Sitting on the couch, reading, or watching TV.

(Probability of stopping = 100 percent. Advice: Keep sitting.)

Want cookies. (Probability of stopping = 90 percent. Advice: Keep sitting, find another TV show or a better book, but don't leave that sofa.)

Walk to kitchen. (Probability of stopping = 75 percent. Advice: Turn around and walk to any other space in the house except the kitchen.)

Get box of cookies. (Probability of stopping = 40 percent. Advice: Put the box down, make some tea, and find an alternative food.)

Open box of cookies. (Probability of stopping = 20 percent. Advice: Put it down, take out just two cookies, and put the box away.)

Start eating cookies. (Probability of stopping = 0 percent. Advice: Don't take the box back with you; limit the number of cookies.)

Take cookies to couch. (Probability of stopping = 0 percent. Advice: Put the box out of your reach.)

Keep eating. (Probability of stopping = 0 percent. Advice: Stop buying cookies.)

Feel sad. (Probability you will do it again = 75 percent. Advice: Stop buying them, or lock them up.)

MINDFUL PERSISTENCE

This book is all about walking away, a trait that society often deems as weak. Persistence, on the other hand, is a strong word; it implies discipline and "stick-to-itiveness." The trick becomes honoring your spider senses and determining when it stops being healthy persistence and when it becomes lazy persistence.

Let's start by talking about quitting. What does this word mean to you? For our purposes, *quitting* is about helplessness and sometimes about exhaustion. Quitting is about not being able to take the long view. Quitting is about not being able to monitor yourself. Quitting is about the belief that you cannot enact the behavioral action—perhaps because you are depleted, don't believe you can do it, or are distracted. What about walking away? *Walking away* is about ownership. It is about knowing that you are done. Walking away is based on data.

Mindless persistence is misguided and often lazy. If we can fall back on an easy golden rule, like "Quitters never win," we are off the hook on doing the true and honest hard work of determining what we really want, listening to ourselves, and thinking about the data. Research on decision-making has shown that when we base our choices and thinking on probabilities, then we are less likely to engage in this sort of blind persistence. Good self-regulation is about mindful *persistence.* We see this at the dinner table and in relationships. The blindness of eating everything on our plate, hungry or not, until the plate is clean is mindless persistence. This mindless persistence can result in unhealthy weight and poor eating habits. The same is true of sticking out relationships that aren't working. Some people may opt to stick it out and give the world a good show, despite knowing that the relationship is kaput. This mindless persistence can result in disrespect, insults, and infidelity. Life is a casino, and after we have incurred losses, sticking it out at the table in hopes that the luck will change to get back "what is ours" can result in throwing bad money after good.

At the dinner table, the blackjack table, or life in general, the trick is to learn when to cut your losses by listening to yourself. True story: I needed a new winter coat for a trip I was taking, I was struggling a bit financially at the time, and I play a decent game of blackjack. So I borrowed some money from my sister, went to a casino in Palm Springs, and I played until I made enough money to buy the damn thing and pay her back. I knew how much I needed exactly ($175), so I played until that cash was in my hands. And then you know what I did? I got up and I walked away. Tempting though it was, I didn't stay, get greedy, or push my luck. I was mindful of my situation (and I still have the coat). Mindful persistence is about seeing something through to a meaningful end point, listening to your spider senses, practicing good gatekeeping, using the data, exercising good communication, and ultimately finding a respectful way to walk away.

Self-regulation, monitoring, and willpower really come down to knowing yourself. You need to stop, quiet down, and listen to yourself. Silence the stakeholders, turn away from the fears, ignore the fairy tales, and realize the conditions under which you work best, what you want, and when you are done. Most of us know what we have to do but we're paralyzed. Self-monitoring can be scary and can feel like listening to demons.

STAYING IN THE MOMENT—EXISTENTIALISM, EATING, AND THE POWER OF HOW

Lots of people these days like to talk about "staying in the moment." It's a nice idea, but a tall order, and one that we don't always understand. In any given moment, you are responsible for your choices. This thought can either be empowering, because you can change the track of your life at every moment, or it can be rather overwhelming, because if you make the wrong choices, it's all on you. If someone else orders your dinner, then you can attack him for making a bad choice; if you order it yourself, those pounds are all you. Many of us talk about mindful eating, and this is really about taking ownership—of your spider senses, and of using attention to remain aware of how stakeholders, fears, and golden rules all work together to keep you eating for everything other than reasons related to food.

One of the key issues in existentialism beyond staying in the present is taking responsibility for your actions. The fact is, *you* put what you put in your mouth. You have the freedom to do what you want, but you have to own it. And it's that second part that people don't like and that makes existentialism a bit of a downer. Eating in a toxic world often leaves us feeling helpless, and I think it is why lots of bad and downright danger-ous diet plans often make so much money. Taking responsibility in the midst of minefields of temptation is difficult. It's for this reason that I am sometimes concerned about the proliferation of weight loss surgery, espe-cially those that are widely advertised such as Lap-Band or gastric bypass. I recognize that in a subset of surgical cases, there is medical necessity. But keep in mind that changing how you eat should be a gradual process that entails learning your preferences, listening to your spider senses, and knowing your body. Weight loss surgeries often outsource that respon-sibility and decision making and change the body without changing the habits or getting rid of the toxic food. Obviously any health-care decision should be made in line with your needs and the consultation of medical professionals, but the more you make this *your* journey and not a path handed down to you from the outside, the greater your chances for suc-cess, not just in weight loss but in all aspects of your life.

This chapter and the remainder of the chapters will discuss how to use staying in the moment and paying attention as ways to address not just eating, but all areas of your life. We now know that a simple choice between a muffin and something healthier, such as fruit, is actually influenced by motivations—both internal and external, rewards both in your brain and from your environment, habits, and whether or not your willpower is depleted. It's a wonder we can make any healthy choices, but we can, and we do.

DECISION-MAKING DILEMMAS

Knowing that our decisions are buffeted by so many forces, both internal and external, it's amazing that we're able to make any choices at all, but we do, dozens of times a day. Remember that the brain is wired for efficiency. We have decision-making systems that are quick and effective (but sometimes wrong), and then we have slower decision-making systems that take into account data (but can also get bogged down in stakeholders and scripts). The power of the pause—just taking a moment—can lift our eating, loving, and living into a mindful space.

EATING IN A TOXIC WORLD

Brains and behavior, dopamine and decision-making, willpower and weakness—these are all very personal, individual processes. But none of this transpires in a vacuum. It all occurs in a context, and that context may feel like a battlefield, given that most of us eat mindlessly and quickly. Add to this the fact that in today's tough economic times, many people are looking for a bargain. We live in a world where the most-rewarding foods (fats, sugars) are the cheapest and easiest to obtain, and they often come in huge portions. It's a perfect storm. Economic problems deplete us and sap our willpower. Cheap food, though it tends to be unhealthy, is frequently served in oversized portions. Stakeholders, fears, and guilt all contribute to fear of waste, which results in less willpower when ordering and eating too much unhealthy food. If you keep eating all the food on your plate or refuse to throw it out because you are trying to be frugal, then, in fact, you are contributing to health problems, and that frugality may end up costing you dearly in health-care costs, unhappiness, sad mood, and poorer health outcomes. Said another way, those $1.00

hamburgers may end up costing you thousands of dollars in health care. This kind of low-priced high-reward food is everywhere—in advertising, vending machines, and drive-through restaurants. When money is tight, making healthy choices can seem like mortal combat. (I recently heard an ad for a place that offered a $6.95 all-you-can-eat pizza lunch, so you can do some "belt loosening instead of belt tightening.") Your spider senses are caught in a David-and-Goliath battle against the world.

When you are depleted, it's difficult to take the long view. Research shows that people without enough economic resources often make more short-sighted decisions, especially with regard to spending, occupational decisions, and health, largely because if they don't have enough, it's hard to look down the road. Consequently, it may feel wrong to "throw away" food today. But if you could manage to take the long view at what these kinds of decisions will cost you in terms of health and wellness, it may no longer feel like "waste."

This is not going to change anytime soon, so while food-policy wonks are doing their thing, you still need to do yours. The world may offer a toxic food environment, but that doesn't mean you can't construct a healthy food environment of your own. You can:

- Clean up your own kitchen and office.
- Identify your stressors and times of depletion.
- Identify the healthy eating options in your community.
- Listen to your spider senses.
- Learn to walk away; just because portion sizes are 30 percent larger doesn't mean you have to be.

THE WHY

Neuroscience and behavioral science provide a way of figuring out what our brains have to say about eating and choice.

- Food is rewarding—in our brains and in our lives.
- It makes us feel good, and it can take away bad feelings, too.
- Willpower can get depleted, and when we are depleted in our brains and bodies, we tend to feel less in control and can end up eating more than we intended.

- When willpower is low, we become shortsighted and don't think about how these bad food choices today may end up costing us money and our health tomorrow.

- Deprivation is not a virtue; in fact, it's a setup for failure.

- Persistence can be a lazy way out; it's time to develop mindful rather than blind persistence.

- Decision-making is vulnerable to lots of influences, and our quick decisions don't always cooperate with our slower decisions.

We are struggling with these challenging decisions in a toxic food environment that bombards us with conflicting images of unrealistic standards of beauty and thinness, along with food pornography. Unless you decide to hide from the world and move to your own farm, you have to find a way to listen to your spider senses and work with your reward-craving brain in a realistic way.

Most of us have been approaching weight management (and likely, life) from the wrong angle. Instead of deprivation and despair, try the magic of mindfulness and monitoring. By simply paying attention, you can work with your brain. And paying attention doesn't need to take much time; it can be just an extra five seconds where you stop and listen before you act.

THE NOW

Retraining your brain takes time. I've provided some exercises that relate to the key concepts in this chapter.

Not Worth the Rewards

Grab your journal and list the ways that food is rewarding for you—and be honest. Taste? Distraction? Makes you feel loved?

List the foods that are most rewarding for you.

Now, make a list of things other than food that are rewarding—again, be honest. Some of these things may be food substitutes (such as shopping); some may be mentally or physically enhancing distractions (walking, reading).

Take this list and post it in the places you go when you are looking for food rewards or distractions. If you are using food as a way to avoid something else, or to "reward" yourself when you are not necessarily hungry, it's time to realize that you can still have rewards in your life—just in a different form.

Willpower

Practice paying attention. Using the tips provided in this chapter—and anything else that works for you—always wait about thirty minutes before diving in. Stop and ask yourself how depleted you are, and reassess your choices. It's time to learn about *repleting* instead of depleting.

We live in a culture where we do everything to extremes. We work too hard, and then we reward ourselves too much. We know that depletion is one of the big willpower killers, so work on finding ways of "repleting" yourself that don't involve food. Some suggestions include:

- exercise,
- a bath or other soothing ritual,
- taking a rest or a nap,
- reading,
- watching a movie or listening to music,
- social connection—in person (ideal), by phone, or online, or
- knitting, painting, or some other creative hobby that you enjoy.

CHECK-IN: BRAINS, BEHAVIOR, AND BAGELS

In your head, create a little gas gauge for yourself to measure your willpower fuel. When are you depleted? When are you weak? What time of day or which situations tap your willpower tank? Awareness might help you drive through your day even if you're on fumes.

CHAPTER 10

Mastering the Cookie Jar— Knowing How to Pull the Triggers

I can resist anything except temptation.

—Oscar Wilde

Give me a person under lock and key and twenty-four hours a day with her, and I can guarantee that I'll get twenty pounds off of her in a month. I can also guarantee that she'll gain back thirty pounds in the next six weeks. On that note, I want to be clear that this book is not about losing weight for your wedding or a special event (a huge mistake, by the way). This book is about taking back your life. This book is about weight management and making sustainable changes, not about losing twenty pounds fast. This is about health at any weight.

What's in your cookie jar at home? Carrots? A big bin of broccoli? No. Cookies. The forbidden and often-hidden treat. Literally or metaphorically, we turn our trigger foods into forbidden fruit, which in turn gives them surplus value. By surplus value I mean foods that are rewarding, or that symbolize celebration or special people or events like grandmothers or cultural traditions. And as we've discussed, when we know something is scarce or special, it makes it difficult to regulate ourselves when we are in the presence of it. In addition, we know that "reward anticipation"—the idea that we are going to get something rewarding (like dessert at the end of a meal)—can start the juices flowing in our brain so that when we are finally faced with the rewarding food, we are actually less able to regulate ourselves in the presence of it.

How often do you feel the desire to binge-drink water? Or blindly eat celery? These are typically not foods that have surplus value, and they are also not rewarding from a brain standpoint. That surplus value tends to come from society. When is the last time you saw an ad for vegetables on TV? Not recently, right? But I'm betting you saw a pizza ad, or ads for something sugary or salty and fried within the last thirty minutes of TV viewing, right?

So, if something is around all the time, it often loses some of its power. I think the same thing can be said for relationships in our lives. We often take for granted those to whom we have regular access. If you completely cut out a food from your life, then your ability to regulate your consumption of it when you get it is often challenging.

There's another dieting practice in our world that I want to warn you about. I am quite leery of services that deliver meals to your home containing exactly the number of calories you need. They tell you exactly what time to eat these meals, and may even give you alarms on your cell phone to alert you. Maybe they tell you how—and how often—to exercise, and exactly how much water to drink in a day. And keep in mind, these services don't come cheap.

You follow it religiously for weeks, or perhaps even months, and you find that you've lost twenty pounds, thirty pounds, forty pounds. But then comes the one-week vacation you take for your friend's wedding. You can't have the food delivered there and you want to have fun. The food is no longer labeled, and golly, that hotel restaurant buffet looks delicious. Since you have been eating out of prepackaged and labeled containers, your gatekeeping skills are shot, and you're out of practice when it comes to your spider senses as well.

Eating a healthy diet and losing weight, especially in the toxic food environments in which we find ourselves, feels impossible, but it's not.

WHAT CONTRIBUTES TO A TOXIC FOOD ENVIRONMENT?

Fast-food restaurants and supersized value meals
All-you-can-eat buffets
Most grocery stores
Convenience stores
Restaurants that serve enormous portions
Vending machines

In the midst of these minefields, we feel like we don't know what to eat, when to eat, and how to eat. With the ensuing frustration, we stop trusting ourselves and put our trust in others. The problem with packaged and structured diet plans is that we outsource all the choice, as well as the responsibility, and in so doing, we also outsource our spider senses.

The problem with packaged and structured diet plans is that we outsource all the choice, as well as the responsibility, and in so doing, we also outsource our spider senses.

WHAT ARE YOUR TRIGGER FOODS?

Let's start by talking about trigger foods. We all have them.

What are they? They are those foods that each of us as individuals find irresistible. Trigger foods taste good, often remind us of a wonderful memory or place, have great texture, and make us feel rewarded. You know you're dealing with a trigger food when you utter an involuntary moan when you eat it.

They are different for all of us, but many times fall under the umbrella of what I call "pleasure" foods: cakes, cookies, sweets, high-fat foods, chips, burgers, pizza, pastries, rich sauces, fried foods, and gourmet offerings. You see or smell them, and before you can even taste them, you know exactly what is coming your way. Some advertisers and food manufacturers bank on this attachment and tap into your trigger. There is even one snack food manufacturer that uses as its slogan "Betcha can't eat just one."

I would like you to take a moment right now and list all of your trigger foods, and I do mean *all* of them. You may add to this list over time. These can be idiosyncratic ones, like your mom's lasagna, your dad's ribs, or your wife's home-baked bread. If you are having trouble, just think about foods that you feel unable to eat less of, foods that make you feel out of control, or foods that frustrate you because you are only supposed to eat one.

I am going to own my list and put myself out there:

- Pizza

- Sandwiches

- Pasta

- Indian food

- Donuts

- Hot dogs

- Eggs Benedict

- Lasagna

- Fried chicken

Once upon a time I couldn't stop myself when I was with these foods. I planned my life around them and rewarded myself with them. That is more power than food should have in a life. Now I use mindfulness and monitoring to help me with these foods. In the course of a year, I may only eat each of these foods once. I make sure that I do not go to them at times when I'm feeling depleted. I tend not to order them, knowing they will find me (at a buffet or a party). When I do get them, I am very careful to portion-control what I get, and share, send away or throw away the rest. But I do have to say this: Instead of being scared of them,

I embrace them. I don't need to eat a bucket of chicken; I can eat one glorious piece, slowly and mindfully, and instead of feeling guilty and out of control, I feel enjoyment.

BREAKING DOWN TRIGGER FOODS

What do you crave?

SUGAR

Sweets cravers are often suckers for sweets across the board. That means they are nondiscriminatory about pies, cakes, cookies, and candies. So if a pie is out, but you're a cupcake person, know you may be just as vulnerable.

Don't substitute. Diet sodas and artificial sweeteners keep you imprisoned by your cravings—be careful there. I know from experience. I am a sweets craver, and go a little too heavy on the diet soda. As a result, I still struggle with self-regulation around sweets.

SALT

Salt cravers will tell you that this craving is just as bad as a sugar craving—and the go-to's here tend to be quick-burn foods like chips and pretzels. These are foods that will often provide an initial carbohydrate boost and then leave the person wanting more. Salty snack foods are also packaged in a way that really plays into mindless eating. If salty foods are your thing, make sure that you don't take the whole big bag, but instead consider keeping smaller-portioned bags of them around. Also consider salty snacks that bring some nutritional bang, such as nuts. (Nuts can also be tricky—they are high in nutrients but also calorie-dense—so just like with anything else, portion them into small bags ahead of time so you don't just blindly eat far more than you intended.)

FAT

Fats can hide in both sweet and salty foods. Most nutrition experts will tell you to consume fats in reasonable quantities. They tend to be calorie-dense, and some fats are easy to over-consume, such as ice cream or fried foods. The basic rule of thumb on things like ice cream: Never eat it directly out of the container. Such foods tend to be very rewarding, and it's extremely difficult to stop after you start eating them. At least if you portion-control them, you have to make a deliberate effort to get more, and if you can use mindfulness and attention at such times, you can stop yourself.

GOURMET

Sometimes we think if food is prepared well at a good restaurant and it's really expensive, it has to be good for us, right? Nope. Rich sauces, fatty meats, and artisanal cheeses have calories, and their presumed virtues and rarity can lead us to eat too much of them. Gourmet triggers are like a fine wine; you should take your time and enjoy them slowly. Recently I went out for a phenomenal dinner with a large group of friends at a gourmet place. Everyone ordered rich pastas, but I was feeling depleted and knew I would eat blindly. I dealt with my gourmet triggers by accepting the tastes offered to me and partaking carefully and mindfully of the exquisite appetizers.

Most trigger foods are rewarding at the level of the brain; I have yet to meet or work with someone who tells me that broccoli is a trigger food. Salad is penance, spaghetti is pleasure. Trigger foods tend to be yummy and rewarding, and they remind us of happy times.

FOOD ADDICTION

If we are trying to manage our weight, trigger foods can be downright scary. We see them and don't feel like we can control ourselves around them. Many diet plans try and take the easy way out and say, just cut out all bad foods. There are endless books out there telling you to cut out refined sugar, fat, high-fructose corn syrup, bread. If you can do that, forever, then I say more power to you. But realistically, most of us find ourselves in places where there are no other options, and I think that instead of eliminating something outright, we are better off learning to consume it. Remember, this even goes back to your stakeholders: You may not be able to cut all of them out of your life entirely, so instead, you need to find a new way to consume them.

When we are told to completely stop eating a food, and then for many reasons we encounter that food, we often find that we do not have the skills to resist it. This is not the same as drugs and alcohol. Here is where food enters a tricky space: When dealing with other addictions like alcohol, tobacco, and drugs, at the end of the day, no one needs those things to survive; we can quit them cold turkey and live a drug- or alcohol-free life. On the other hand, we have to eat, and we're faced with dozens of food choices each day. Just being told to say no is not preparing us for difficult times. One tricky bit with the trigger foods is something called the "abstinence violation effect," first postulated by alcohol researcher Alan Marlatt. It's a fancy way of saying "falling off the wagon." Basically once a person "slips" and eats the forbidden food, he or she will say "to hell with it, I screwed up my diet so I might as well eat the whole thing." A similar pattern is seen in recently abstinent alcoholics.

Having two forkfuls of cheesecake, especially if you know how to eat cheesecake, is not your demise; in fact, it may be your salvation. By having just a couple of forkfuls, you learn a lesson: You can tolerate a trigger food without feeling out of control. But finding this middle ground means breaking rules. You have to defy the legion of stakeholders who feel you are wasting food when you don't finish the entire portion, or defying golden rules about clean plates, or facing fears of "not having enough food later," or fears of letting people down because you didn't clean your plate after they cooked for hours.

Life is short. Do you really want to spend the rest of your life never partaking of foods that give you pleasure again? I don't think so. It's about learning to consume them properly, and about finding pleasure in the many other places in life where it also exists.

In this book there are no forbidden foods; I don't care what you eat, and at no point am I going to put out a prescriptive guide to eating. There are many books that already do that, and the fact is, you know the answers already. All of us know how to eat, but knowing and doing are two different things. Most theories of health behavior will tell you that knowledge doesn't predict behavior—things like attitudes do. So change your attitude about these trigger foods and then you'll be able to change your behavior.

MANAGING TRIGGER FOODS

Start simple: *Don't order trigger foods,* because they will come to you. When you are on your own and making the decisions, simply don't order them. Use your alone times to make optimal decisions. Usually celebrations and other people will bring trigger foods into our lives. You will expend enough effort to manage them there, so don't bring them in voluntarily. This also means that you shouldn't bring them into your kitchen. If the cookies aren't in the kitchen, you won't go and grab them. If they need to be in your kitchen, then put them in a cabinet with a child lock. The extra minute it takes you to fool with the lock should be a moment when you say to yourself, "Really?"

If you do order them yourself, throw out half right away. Especially with a trigger food, don't be shy about throwing them away. For example, sometimes at a birthday party or wedding, the cake is cut and brought to you. It's okay to eat just half or a few forkfuls and then leave the rest. Don't worry; nobody will notice, and if they do, so what? Answer only to yourself.

When they come to you, partake sparingly. If you can break off half the cookie, or cut the pie or burger to a manageable size, do so right out of the gate. If you are eating with someone else, share the other half. If it's sitting in front of you, the temptation is hard to fight.

Don't take home the leftovers. Ever. This is a tough one because it feels wasteful. Restaurants give you too much food, and with trigger foods, if they're at home you'll follow them into the fridge late at night for another hookup. Just because the calories are eaten at two different times doesn't mean they don't add up.

Eat trigger foods slowly. Make love to that cheesecake. Put a small forkful in your mouth. Roll it on your tongue. Really enjoy it. We tend to eat trigger foods too quickly and blindly, ignoring our spider senses and letting the decision-making go out the window because it is so rewarding. So slow down, and much like sex, prolong the pleasure. A 100-calorie portion can be just as rewarding as a 1,000-calorie brick of cake if you eat it slowly. Then when you are done, you can not only revel in the pleasure of the cheesecake, but also the satisfaction of having listened to and regulated yourself.

Try the paradoxical prescription. Do you have a trigger food that you both crave and fear? Force yourself to eat a 100-calorie portion of it every day. When I have patients with triggers they feel as though they will panic if they can't have it, or that they'll go out of control when they do, so we build it into their daily lives. Over time it loses much of its power.

Fix the context. If bread is your trigger and your dining companions are amenable, then ask the waiter not to bring any bread. Our danger is in grabbing at trigger foods blindly; if they aren't there to grab, then you'll be okay. That also means keeping them out of your house, car, desk, and purse.

If you don't learn to coexist with the cookie jar, the cookie jar will own you. Instead, invite it in on your own terms.

USE YOUR BRAIN

People love being told what to do because it's easier and requires less responsibility, less listening to ourselves, and less struggle. Diet books that tell you exactly what to eat, at what time, and in what quantity are successful because they allow you to shut off your mind and not take full ownership of what you are doing. Take, for example, the ones that allow for all the cheese and oil and fat you want, as long as you don't eat a single grain or starch. This is simply not sustainable for most people. By blindly following, you're not listening to your body, and in essence you're outsourcing your spider senses. It also makes it hard to eat with other people. But, here's the part people love: When it doesn't work, it can be written off to the plan, which is easier and less scary than taking responsibility for your own weight gain.

SURVIVING TRICKY SITUATIONS

Just know, I never said this would be easy, but there are some tricks you can employ to get you through the most difficult situations, because life simply happens and you will encounter them no matter how much you work to survive. And for yourself, when you come across a situation that trips you up, make a note, mental or actual. Figure out a way to blast through it without derailing all that you've worked to achieve.

The Buffet

Buffets are the death knell for people trying to manage weight, and yet they are perceived as having such value in our bargain-obsessed society. If we are at a buffet, we feel like we have to get our "money's worth," and therefore we overeat. In general, buffets are priced so that they seem like a better bargain in terms of dollars per pound of food than a la carte, and from a strict dollars-and-cents perspective, they are. But that's where the bargain begins and ends.

The way many buffet days go down for people are as follows: Some folks feel like they "deserve" the buffet as a reward after a hard week of work, and so they just eat with abandon. It is easy to consume 3,000 to 4,000 calories at a buffet in a single sitting. Some people try to be strategic buffet eaters: Oooh, we are going to that fabulous buffet brunch / all-you-can-eat restaurant / salad buffet restaurant later today, so I better "be good" today; I may even go to the gym, and then I am only going to eat good stuff and restrict what I eat so I can eat anything I want later. Remember what Baumeister and many other researchers say about willpower: We often don't have enough willpower to go around, and the many choices at a buffet can leave us unable to make good choices, so we don't make any—we just eat what we want. If you go to a buffet having restricted yourself all day and having used up all of your willpower, you will likely binge.

Buffets are like a war zone for your spider senses. We typically go in wanting to get our money's worth, being terrible gatekeepers and putting too much on our plates, feeling compelled to finish them, and joining in with our stakeholders. This is a dietary disaster waiting to happen. I faced down a buffet the other day when a hotel made an error in my bill. To make amends they offered me lunch. I was alone and the only place to eat was a brunch buffet. It was not for the faint of heart. I literally felt anxious as I stared down the table filled with breakfast meats, muffins, cakes, pies, and a crepe station. It was the first buffet I had encountered in about twelve months. I was reminded that all-you-can-eat setups are never a good idea. I took a deep breath, tasted some tricky favorites, indulged in the fresh fruits and vegetables, and felt no compunction about leaving a little behind.

Parties and Family Gatherings

These kinds of events are killers; not only are they filled with trigger foods, but they can also be viewed as "trigger events." We have to attend—and thus, survive—them, and if we learn to listen to our spider senses, we may even thrive in them. Beating the challenge of trigger events often seems impossible. Some families or communities are just focused on having lots of good food all the time, and certain jobs can require attendance at frequent food-heavy events. On such days you don't want to over-deprive on the front end, so you wind up making bad decisions later. Eat breakfast on these days, so you are able to engage in your mindfulness minute and good gatekeeping. These events, particularly family gatherings, can bring up strong (and sometimes unpleasant) emotions, which we try to avoid by eating. And, if ever there were a situation in which to say this: Watch out for those stakeholders. In some families not eating the pie is no different than slapping your aunt or grandmother across the face.

TRICKS FROM SOMEONE WHO KNOWS

Take the pie and eat it slowly, enjoying only a few bites. When Grandma is distracted, ditch the rest without hurting her feelings.

Stay away from the food if it's set out on a table for self-serve. If it is sit-down, when the meal is done and it's appropriate to do so, get out of there and go to another area and continue conversations there.

If you have a choice of taking your food and moving away from the serving plates, do it! Avoid the "snatch and grab" reflexive food grabs that can translate into hundreds of under-the-radar calories. If you indulge ten times in the trays of tiny 100-calorie bites being walked around, you've racked up some calories, and that will undo you.

Eat for You

I was recently in a restaurant in New York. I was cold and craving the crepes they had in the window—even though I knew full well that an entire crepe contained too much sugar, fat, and calories. I just wanted about one-third of one, but they would not make that for me. So I ordered the whole thing, ate the three or four forkfuls I wanted, was completely satisfied, and then I was done. The waitress looked ashen when she came to check on me, and I asked her to take it away. She said, "Wasn't it good?" I am a pleaser and I felt sad for her. In fact, the crepe was delicious, but I didn't want to eat the entire thing. I could easily have seen where her reaction and my drive to please would have led me to eat more, to show her that I liked it. Instead, I relied on my words to communicate for me. I told her it was fantastic, and that I'd had exactly as much as I wanted. She wasn't convinced, but it wasn't my job to convince her; I got exactly what I wanted. I didn't order or eat the crepe to please her; I got it for me. I've had this same experience during dinner at people's homes, and eating out in a number of venues. If you don't finish, you feel like you're letting someone down, or that somehow, your eating is coming under scrutiny. The fear of letting someone down is one of our most primitive fears. Stand your ground, especially where trigger foods are concerned.

DISTRACT DESIRE WITH DESIRE, NOT DEPRIVATION

Keep in mind that the more you spend down your willpower, the less of it you will have. So don't always face down food desires with deprivation. Instead, substitute them with something else you desire. I have a friend who is a writer, so she works from home. I told her to satisfy other desires in order to avoid the munchies. She was craving a midday snack but had already eaten her snack for the afternoon. She was struggling because she knew she wanted to scratch her itch, and she'd been working so hard at losing weight. She decided to take a break and indulge in her other obsession: watching TV. She had some shows recorded that she was saving for the weekend, but knowing she was fidgety for food, she went to the TV and indulged in some workday viewing. She didn't eat again until dinnertime, and felt like she'd had a luxurious treat anyway.

We can't always do what we want to do; that's life. Because we can't always do what we want to do, and food is available to just about all of us as a quick reward, we often use it. If we are idle eaters that start grabbing the goodies because we feel deprived, depleted, or otherwise despondent, we tend to have a trigger that we abuse. We need to learn to rely on other things that are pleasurable, and easier to regulate.

CALORIE-FREE PLEASURE

Make a list of escapist pleasures and go to them instead:

- Take a bath.

- Take a walk.

- Read a book.

- Fiddle around on Facebook.

- Have sex or even masturbate (depending on whether you're at home or work or in traffic) when the munchies hit. It's pleasurable, distracting, and often after an orgasm, you may not feel as hungry.

Structure Your Environment

We need to create a balance between temptation and temperance, and these tips are focused on ways to create that balance:

Clean out the minefield. Remove or minimize the triggers in your home—the candy or chips. Walk to the store and buy a single-serving bag and enjoy it instead of buying the family-size bag and eating the entire thing.

Lock the cupboards if you need to. I actually put child locks on my cabinets and a little Post-it by the lock, asking "Is it worth it?" Sometimes the momentary delay to fudge with the child lock gave me pause to stop and ask myself if I was eating because I was frustrated, lonely, anxious, or bored (my usual reasons for eating), and then I redirected those emotions.

Putting trigger snacks in the freezer works sometimes, too. We tend not to go to the freezer as often, so we can experience the "out of sight, out of mind" element. But some people may actually enjoy frozen snack foods better, so make sure it doesn't make them more appealing!

Keep food in food spaces. I have had patients who had refrigerators in their bedrooms, cookies in their nightstands, and candy in their cars.

When you can't do the quick grab, you are less likely to get into trouble. If you are going to keep a few things with you to take the edge off when you are really hungry, keep the healthy options close by.

One tool that helped me immeasurably with my weight loss was to bring my own lunches to work (I can control the portions better), and to bring a variety of fresh fruits and vegetables in on Monday, as well as some multigrain bars and other options for times I needed a grab-and-go snack between classes. I was fortunate because the nearest place to purchase food was a five- to seven-minute walk away, and by ensuring that the easy reach was healthy, I made fewer food mistakes. It's like grocery shopping when you're hungry; if you head to a place to buy lunch when you're starving, you might choose incorrectly, but if, when your stomach growls, your healthy lunch is already on your desk, you're in better shape.

If there is a snack food you like, portion it out ahead of time and put it in little bags. If you try to do that for yourself from a larger bag, trust me, you will overestimate.

The Grocery Store

Grocery stores are minefields, and the people who put the food in the store use marketing science to draw you in and get you to buy—and not necessarily the good stuff. Use all the strategies that you can, like not shopping when you're hungry or depleted because your willpower won't be as strong in the face of those giant packages of cookies. And just like you can use a smaller plate to cut down on eating, you can also use a smaller cart to cut down on loading it up. When possible, consider using a hand carried basket instead of a cart (I realize that this is not always possible if you are shopping for a big family or stocking up) but try it and see how you choose when you can't make impulse buys. Sometimes the smaller basket makes you more mindful and forces you to take that extra moment to stop and think instead of blindly throwing the items in your cart. Remember, if it doesn't come into the house, you are less likely to eat it. I sometimes try a fun technique at one of my favorite local grocery stores—I don't use a cart or a basket, only purchase what I can carry in my hands, and invariably I actually make better choices and am able to tell myself no. In the shopping chapter I will also talk about avoiding the big box stores where the big bargains can lead to even bigger weight gain.

Here are some other tips to help you more gracefully handle the triggers in the grocery store.

- Make a list and stick to it.

- If you live in a major metropolitan area, there are grocery delivery services that allow you to order groceries online and then get them delivered. You may be less likely to make impulse purchases if you don't smell and see the food.

- Don't get drawn in by the "stock-up" deals or bulk items. Then the stuff is in the house and you eat it.

- Read labels. Calories and sugar lurk in odd places (yogurt can seem like a healthy option but some brands contain lots of sugar, and "fat-free" foods can be calorie laden).

- Remember how prior generations shopped, and how many parts of the world still do. If you have the luxury to do so, try to shop more regularly for fresher ingredients and steer away from the processed stuff. Our parents often went to the butcher, baker, and market daily to prepare dinner. I realize that modern schedules can make this tough though, and I am very guilty of relying on the pre-prepared stuff more than I should. But I do know that whenever I walk into a grocery, that night, my girls and I tend to eat more freshly prepared stuff than when I do not.

STRATEGIES FOR EATING OUT

Restaurants are where healthy eating often goes to die. We can't control the ingredients, portion sizes, side dishes, stakeholders, and so on. But it is also a big part of our culture, and frankly, it's fun. Eating out is all about planning and mindfulness. Restaurants don't have to be danger zones, but rather places where you need to let your spider senses in, be fearless about walking away, and not get caught up in pleasing others.

Course by Course

One of my favorite sushi places in Los Angeles is called Sugarfish. It is the single diner's fantasy restaurant. Many times eating out alone is a nuisance, because you may not give in to the multiple steps (or calories) of ordering appetizer and entree, and as such may also be limited in terms of variety. When you order one thing, you eat it, and before you know it, you've finished. Sugarfish has a series of price-fixed menus (some as low as about 400 calories), and they pace the meal nicely. Even with so few calories, it comes out in four courses, each presented beautifully. The amount of food isn't that much, but the pacing and the quality of the food leaves you feeling taken care of and full.

Eat in phases. We tend to put everything in front of us at once and then eat it all at once. For anyone who has ever celebrated Christmas, or a birthday or other "gift-y" holiday, you know how it feels: You have a big pile of gifts in front of you, and after opening them all, you often feel numb and dejected. Do you remember how good it felt when a few more gifts were pulled out later, or if you opened the gifts over a longer period of time? Meals are similar. If you can serve or eat the meal in phases—eat one thing (such as a salad) and let it breathe, and then eat something else—even if the portions are very small, it's a celebratory way to eat and prolongs the eating experience.

Harness Hotness

It's interesting that in English when we ask if food is hot, it can mean temperature or spice. Telugu, the language I grew up with, actually has two food-temperature words: one that means spicy heat, and another that means temperature heat. That being said, if I only learned one thing growing up with hot spicy, food, it's that it slows us down when we're eating it. I was raised on Indian food that was hot in terms of both temperature and spice, and this often slows me down significantly, which typically results in my being aware that I am full and being able to eat less yet still feel satisfied.

THE WHY

Invite your trigger foods in, and by using tools such as the mindfulness minute, monitoring, portion control, restructuring your environment, and being good to yourself with things other than food, you can exist in a toxic food world and honor yourself.

The fact is, trigger foods are everywhere, and they are powerful. It is not realistic to think that you can construct a world where they do not exist. It's also not realistic to take on a diet plan that eliminates "bad foods." There are no bad foods—just bad decisions.

THE NOW

Here's an exercise that I really want you to consider carefully. For your next meal or snack, put a plate of something really tempting in front of you. Then, take a mindfulness minute and prepare yourself to be with the food. Now, eat only half of it. Throw the rest of it in the garbage.

- Write down how you felt.

- Was it a challenge?

- Was it easy?

- After you were done with your half of the plate, were you still hungry?

You can practice this a few ways over time. In my experience people are extremely resistant to this exercise; the clean-plate club is a heavy childhood lesson, and people feel there is some sort of horror in waste. Since you cannot control how the world serves food, you want to use good gatekeeping as often as possible so you can learn to take the proper amount, eat it mindfully, and feel satisfied. These exercises let you exert some dirty-plate muscle:

At home, use cookies. Put four on the plate. Eat two and toss two.

Order in. Scoop the appropriate portion size onto the plate and throw the rest in the garbage.

At the restaurant, before you even cut into the food, ask for a second plate, divide the portion in half, and hand the waiter the other half.

Now for the trickiest part of this, employ two witnesses or stakeholders and do it in front of them. See how they react. Will they say, Are you sure?

CHECK-IN: TRIGGER FOOD SPEED BUMP

When faced with trigger foods, create for yourself a speed bump in the road. When you see cake on someone's desk, before you accept a piece, count to ten; or, choose a word and say it out loud, like "Stop." Whatever it is, and however you react afterward, make sure you hit that bump in your road first before you mindlessly indulge.

CHAPTER 11

Quit the Clean-Plate Club

Part of the secret of success in life is to eat what you like
and let the food fight it out inside.

—Mark Twain

Here is the current state of knowledge and advice on weight loss in the
world today:

- Eat less.
- Exercise more.
- Eat healthier.
- Don't eat junk food.

Ask anyone on the street what a healthy meal looks like and how to
lose weight, and they will give you a perfect answer. But knowledge is
not behavior, and despite knowing all of this, we live in a country where
one-third of adults are obese.

SIMPLE SOLUTIONS TO A COMPLEX PROBLEM

Let's take those four points one by one, since they form the foundation
of what is supposed to be a successful weight-management routine. They
are not the whole shooting match—they're just the basic principles—but
take all that you've learned in this book and combine it with these four
points, and you will defeat your food issues.

Eat Less

Your spider senses are essential in the ongoing battle with weight loss. This is about brain, environment, motivation, willpower, our personal histories, our stakeholders, and our lifestyles. This is about monitoring and mindfulness. On one weight-loss show on which I worked, a client looked at his 400-calorie lunch, which had been carefully portioned and served in a tiny little take-out container. A wonderful mélange of chicken, rice, and vegetables, it appeared small in terms of volume. He said he literally felt "panicky" at the beginning of the meal that he wouldn't have enough to eat. But by eating slowly, and enjoying each bite, he found he was satisfied at the end of the meal.

We tend to eat so quickly that small meals can feel scary, and if we look at the meal right out of the gate and think it won't be enough, our brains can make us feel like it isn't. Instead, enjoy each bite. It's not simply a matter of eating less; it's also about listening to our spider senses and being mindful of when we are full so that we don't consume huge portions.

PORTION SIZES

The National Institutes of Health reveals that portion sizes have increased anywhere from 30 to 100 percent, depending on the food, in the past twenty years, and since we love to clean our plates, you do the math. So even when there is triple the amount of food on the plate than you'd normally eat, you feel compelled to finish it. (In the resources section at the end of this book you'll find links to some visually compelling data comparing portion sizes twenty years ago with now.)

LET YOUR MIND PLAY TRICKS

Remember, I don't care what you eat. This is about a lifelong new approach to food—one that involves using food for nutrition and listening to your body and mind in all areas of your life. But there are a few tricks you can practice to make eating less a little easier. First, it's time for you to get new plates. In my home we no longer use dinner plates; we use bread plates for dinner. And what are often being sold as dinner plates could actually suffice quite nicely as serving platters. If you are staring at a huge plate that looks empty, you will automatically feel deprived before you ever start eating. Over the past few years, they've been making plates larger than they used to, keeping up with those ever-growing portion sizes. I have found smaller plates at a variety of vendors, and you can choose fun shapes and colors. Restaurant owners tend to use enormous plates, enormous glasses, and enormous utensils, but at home if you make them smaller, you will eat less and slow down. Interestingly, in parts of the world where obesity and being overweight are not nearly as endemic (e.g. Western Europe), coffee cups, plates, and bowls are significantly smaller.

Second, if you want to eat less, eat more slowly. Our brain needs a minute to catch up. If you just shove in a bunch of food, it needs a second to say, "Oh, I'm full." We know that we are terrible at heeding our signals that we are full. So by eating slowly, you will eat less. Here is where we return to monitoring, attention, and not eating while distracted. Often when we do something else, we eat faster. Make eating about eating.

MINDLESS EATING

A recent study conducted by Brian Wansink and his colleagues points out how mindlessly we can eat. Two groups were given different situations. One group had a normal bowl of soup that would empty out as they ate it. The other group had specially designed bowls that had a pump system built into the bottom that could add more soup to the bowl as the person ate (they were not aware of this). Everyone was told to stop eating when they were full. The people who had the bowls that kept refilling ate 73 percent more before reporting they were full than those who had the regular bowls of soup, supporting the assertion that we often use visual cues to figure out if we are full (clean plates), rather than our true feeling of fullness. As such, trying to fill our plates with the right amount of food, eating slowly, and then giving our minds a chance to catch up with our stomachs is key.

Remember what we talked about in the previous chapter—spreading out the "courses" to make eating more special? There's a little mental trick with that strategy as well. Many people feel like smaller portion sizes equal less time eating. Eating is in fact pleasurable, so it's not just about consuming food, but also about consuming time. By breaking the meal into smaller plates and phases, you prolong it and give your brain and gut (and spider senses) a chance to kick in and stop you from overeating. This also may reinforce eating more slowly.

Exercise More

Fitness experts and aficionados will freak out over this next section, but nutritionists will wholeheartedly agree. I want to be clear: To get your weight under control, you need to control your eating and generally your psychological approach to food intake. People who have a weight issue and assume they can exercise it off are misled, and will waste a lot of time thinking they can eat whatever they want as long as they hit the gym. It's completely false.

From a strictly mathematical and efficiency perspective, exercise as a weight-loss "tool" doesn't really make sense. While you can spend an hour on a treadmill huffing and puffing and maybe knock out 600 to 800 calories, you can probably turn around and consume that many calories in about five to eight minutes with a tuna sandwich and some coleslaw. So while exercise may aid in weight loss, it will only work if you also change your eating patterns. You can't allow an intense workout to justify eating whatever you want. When people exercise, it begets hunger, and many people assume that the exercise is a get-out-of-jail-free card: I worked out, so I can eat anything I want. But the truth is, you can't. There are 3,500 calories in a pound. If you burn that many, you lose a pound. If you burn 600 calories in a workout and then eat a 1,200-calorie lunch (that you would not have eaten had you not worked out), then you are wasting your time and fighting a losing battle.

The other problem is that often people "go to the gym" and phone it in. If you can read or talk while you exercise, you are probably not burning nearly as many calories as you think.

That said, exercise is essential—not for weight loss, but for vitality and health. This isn't a book about losing weight; this is a book about living a full, authentic, and healthy life. Exercise enhances your spider senses because it puts you in better touch with your body. I am a firm believer in health and beauty at any weight. Recent studies show that if you lose weight, the key to keeping it off is exercise. Even more important, exercise boosts cardiovascular and immune function, bone and joint health, muscle tone, and cognitive function. It helps you to manage stress and a host of chronic illnesses, like diabetes, and may have protective benefits for mental health issues, including depression and anxiety. The list is endless.

Again, listen to yourself and not your stakeholders. Don't feel like you have to run five miles every day just because that's what your best friend did to lose weight. You will only wind up frustrated and demoralized. Instead, find something you really enjoy—whether it's playing a game of tennis or attending a yoga class. If you hate the gym, don't force yourself to go. Find something more in line with your spider senses, such as taking a walk outside.

Exercise can help tweak your metabolism, and it may be as close to a cure-all as anything else that we have in our health toolbox. And yes, it can help you manage your weight. My point is that exercise alone is not the key; in fact, it ranks low compared to how you approach food and learn to pay attention to yourself whenever you eat. At the end of the day, if you want to lose or manage weight, eat less.

Eat Healthier

I am not a dietitian or nutritionist, and this book is not about *what* to eat; it's about why you eat. The choices you make in terms of healthfulness are related to the themes of this book. Feed yourself as if you were your own child. When you make unhealthy choices, think about whether that is how you would feed someone you really care about. You are a finely tuned machine, so treat yourself as such. If you had a really expensive car that needed expensive gas, you would probably take the time and money to fill it properly so that it would run better, so why would you treat yourself any differently?

FAKING IT—SUGAR SUBSTITUTES

Folks like Linda Bartoshuk, a psychologist and professor at the University of Florida who studies taste and obesity, and Susan Swithers and Terry Davidson, psychologists at Purdue, have talked about the link between taste and weight. Swithers and Davidson have conducted animal studies on artificial sweeteners, and guess what. That saccharine trickery may not be working. They postulate that when we drink diet sodas, our brain gets the signal of "sweet" but our bodies don't get the glucose. They believe that the brain uses taste as an index of the calories to come, which we then need to burn. When the actual calories don't follow the taste, what may happen is eating more or burning less energy. In their studies, the rats that ate saccharine-sweetened food gained more weight. When our brains get the sweet signal it maintains our sugar cravings and throws off our brain and body's ability to manage our energy demands. Artificial sweeteners are like methadone is to heroin—meant to get us off of sugar without the caloric effects—but the original problem of craving "sweet" remains, and we continue to struggle with the craving. Watch your patterns with artificial sweeteners and see if you kick it up at certain times, because it may be setting you up for even bigger sugar transgressions at other times in the day and for weight gain down the road.

CHOOSE HEALTHY FOODS

Healthier foods such as fruits, vegetables, lean proteins, and multigrain products tend to stay with us longer so we don't fall prey to the hunger bug.

Make healthy food a habit. If that's all you have around and you're hungry, you will reach for it.

Make your plate colorful. Half of your plate should be vegetables and fruits.

This is about respect and honoring your body. It is shortsighted to consistently choose the unhealthy option. Each time you choose the less-than-healthy option, wait a beat and think about what you are about to put into your body. Choose well. When you eat well-prepared food made with high-quality ingredients, a little goes a long way. The more you learn to listen to—and honor—yourself, the more it will extend to how you feed yourself.

LIQUID LUNCH

Watch the liquids. I recently worked with a patient who assumed that when you drink calories, they don't count as much. A calorie is a calorie whether it comes from a carrot or candy. Drinking rich coffee drinks, sports drinks, and sodas can push 500 to 800 calories into your day without you even thinking about it. Those "frappy" drinks at your coffee shop can pack a 400- to 600-calorie wallop. We often drink more mindlessly than we eat, so we ingest those calories without even thinking about it. Also, be careful of going to those juice stores; you may think you're drinking a cup of fruit, but a large one of those can put you back 400 calories or more, and again, we often consume them more mindlessly, and they often do not leaving us feeling as satisfied so we are hungry more quickly.

Don't Eat Junk Food

Junk food and fast food are the demise of most of us—fast, cheap, accessible, tasty, and rewarding. As with all things, moderation is the order of the day, and sometimes junk food is thrust upon us on a road trip, in an airport, or at a kid's party. If you do eat junk, at least listen to your spider senses and walk away when you are full. The world makes it hard to eat well, but you can do it by remaining mindful and heeding your spider senses. Pizza is not inherently bad; it's all about portion size. You know that eating an entire pizza is unhealthy, so don't do it. One slice? Bon appétit!

Feed yourself as if you were your own child. When you make unhealthy choices, think about whether that is how you would feed someone you really care about.

Every meal is an opportunity to make new and healthier choices. And if you didn't quite hit the healthy target at your last meal, don't fret; your next meal is a chance to get it right.

HOW TO AVOID CLEAN-PLATE MISTAKES IN A DIRTY-FOOD PORN WORLD

So many of my clients believe deprivation means they are "doing weight loss right." They can usually pull it off for a few weeks, maybe even a few months. They sometimes say that the feeling of hunger makes them feel virtuous. Some even build in "cheat days." I hate that term, as though you were doing something immoral with a bowl of pasta. The so-called cheat days are viewed as the exception, and they are often a dysregulated mess—a day when the person is finally back with the food they want, and after a week of steamed vegetables and skinless chicken, they embrace that pasta like a lover's kiss after a long absence.

I firmly believe in inviting the demons to the table at every meal. Demons get their power by sitting in the darkness where they can taunt us. When you invite them out, they lose a lot of that power. Instead of "cheat days," bring the foods you like into every meal and learn to be with them in a reasonable way. One slice of pizza with that salad. Half the sandwich and the vegetable soup. The great Chinese food dish, skipping the rice. Half the brownie with your tea. Listening to your spider senses and feeding yourself should not be illicit or forbidden, and it doesn't mean you're a failure. Let the scary foods in.

So once you decide to invite those scary foods in, I want you to go to a restaurant and order that slice of cheesecake or bowl of bisque. The problem is that the restaurants are often not on the same page (or plate) as you. Their patrons expect big servings, and they may lose customers with small portion sizes. Large portion sizes don't cost them that much more, but they keep customers coming back. Go to a restaurant, but try to eat an appropriate portion. In a world of large portion sizes, you need to use your spider senses to inform good gatekeeping.

So you order that forbidden food but are now given an inappropriately large serving size. Ignore the childhood teaching to clean your plate. This book is all about the dirty-plate club, not the clean-plate club we learned about when we were four. What do we do in the dirty-plate club? We walk away when we are done. We ignore our stakeholders. We shelve the fears. We give up the childhood myths. We listen to ourselves.

So when you are eating outside of your house, try these tips to get you there:

- Ask your server if he will bring you a smaller portion (ideally the restaurant will charge you less, but they may not). If he will cut the portion, then great. And stop fretting about how you didn't get your money's worth. If half of that eight-ounce cup of bisque filled you up and gave you pleasure, then you just got your money's worth.

- If your server can't bring you a smaller portion, then ask for a smaller plate or bowl, create your portion size right there, and make her take away the rest immediately. That unfinished portion will keep staring at you with a come-hither look, and if you are feeling depleted or want a reward, you may just start blindly eating. Take away the trigger.

- Keep the context clean. Try to avoid classic mistakes like having the serving plates at the table, because it is too easy to go for seconds. Keeping the plates at the table can scramble your spider senses, because you may not take that mindfulness minute to ask yourself if you are actually still hungry.

- Cut it down to size: Order the smaller size even if it doesn't seem as "economical."

- Stop buying for an army. Avoid shopping at big-box stores and bringing home all those large quantities that you will then feel compelled to consume.

- Say goodbye to the buffet. Even if the buffet breakfast seems like a better deal, order a la carte. You will eat less.

- Share the food. If you are dining with friends or a companion, each of you can order one thing and then split it. It gives you a greater variety of flavors, and you may eat less as a result.

- Watch the wine. Alcohol has calories, but more important, alcohol also lowers our filters and can impair decision-making. We are less able to pay attention, monitor, and allow our spider senses to work if we are numbed by alcohol. Take it nice and slow and try to eat before you drink too much.

THE MEDICAL FINE PRINT

Dietary and activity changes of any kind should be undertaken after getting clearance from your health-care professional. You should consider the tips below if you are going to embark on a program of changes in what you eat and how you exercise: Resources and websites for those seeking further assistance are also provided at the end of the book.

1. See your physician to review any issues related to medications, lab results, or existing health conditions before changing your diet, using supplements of any kind, or starting an exercise program.

2. Consider seeking out therapy with a licensed mental health professional if through this process you find that longer–term psychological issues may be significantly impacting how you eat and live.

3. If you are feeling out of control with food, either controlling what you eat too much, losing significant amounts of weight, or engaging in behaviors to get rid of food (purging, using laxatives, excessive exercise), see a health-care professional as soon as possible.

THE WHY

When you reflect on how to eat, you need to start with why you eat. And when you are faced with those whys, be able to stop, look, listen, and then act. Eating less, exercising more, eating healthier, and not eating junk food will only get you so far. You also need to trust your spider senses and be mindful of how you are treating your body.

THE NOW

This is more like homework than an exercise. I want you to change your eating by fixing your environment. We have already reviewed much of this, but practice makes perfect, and these small fixes can lead to big changes.

Start with investing in some small plates. I buy rice bowls in Chinatown and use them for cereal—that way I'm not tempted to over-pour into a typical bowl. Observe the difference once you switch them out. Are you satisfied? Are you noticing a change in how much you consume?

Start reading labels to learn portion sizes and then use measuring cups to measure at home. That way you can't lie to yourself about what's on the plate. A half a cup of rice is okay; two cups is not (even if it is brown). Use the resources listed in the back of the book to get a handle on portion sizes.

Purge your home. Clean out your cabinets and desk at work, and toss out the foods that are dangerous for you. Let the junk find you, but don't invite it in. I have a patient who likes nuts, and I'm fine with her eating them. But instead of buying a ten-pound bag and parking it in her kitchen to taunt her, she treats herself once a week to a one-serving bag full when she attends a weekly writing class.

Order small. Get into the habit of ordering the smallest size offered.

If fear was a part of your childhood dinner table, think of ways you can reconfigure this. Many times a kitchen table can be an anxious place because of your early lessons. You can reconfigure the table and change or rotate who sits at the head of your table, encouraging conversation. Avoid putting the serving platters on the table, so fear doesn't lead you to eat blindly.

CHECK-IN: CLEAN DIRTY PLATE

When you're eating with other people, watch them. Some are indifferent to food, while others shovel it in so quickly it actually hurts your chest. Sometimes, it will make you more mindful about how you eat, and more aware of things you might do that you didn't even realize until you saw the habit in someone else.

PART THREE:

Eating Patterns = Life Patterns

CHAPTER 12

Food as Metaphor

One cannot think well, love well, and sleep well, if one has not dined well.

—Virginia Woolf

Ms. Woolf nailed it: We must take care of ourselves and nourish ourselves if we are going to be able to regulate ourselves in other parts of our lives. Food is our first lesson in self-regulation, and all of our other self-regulation lessons stem from our relationship with food and our ability to adjust it. This chapter introduces the next section in the book, showing how food can serve as a metaphor, and why your relationship with food impacts love, life, work, and so many other things.

When I lost the weight, I did not use a trainer, nutritionist, surgery, or pills. People asked me, "What did you do?" I usually kept it short and replied, "I changed what I ate and exercised more." Over time I felt more and more uncomfortable with that answer, because it wasn't true. The right answer was: I took myself seriously, I said no to people, I got the junk out of my house, I learned to walk away from half-full plates and bad situations, I made some painful decisions regarding my marriage, and I took risks. And because of that, I took care of myself and subsequently lost weight. Most important—I finally listened to myself and lived life in accordance with my spider senses.

This is not about avoiding soda, or doing 300 abdominal crunches every morning, or eliminating carbohydrates from your diet. This is not about eating lean fish and avoiding certain kinds of meats and always ordering sauce on the side. These things may help, but these things alone will not bring you to a place of health. They are the battle, but they are absolutely not the war. In some ways this is about hope—about envisioning a future, and not being afraid of failing, but being afraid of not trying. For every meal that you make some bad choices, there are some where you make good ones. Be kind to yourself and see how right you are able to get it.

When I looked at the evidence from the field of psychology, medicine, nutrition, and exercise physiology, the answer was simple: Weight management is about something much bigger than what you eat for breakfast. But why and how you eat speaks volumes about how you live your life.

There is no greater metaphor for how we regulate ourselves in every aspect of our lives than eating, partly because we do it multiple times a day. Eating is an example of how we are able to listen to ourselves (or not), and how much we are able to weigh what we need and want against the voices of stakeholders, fears, and the golden rules of our youth. Our eating habits give us powerful insight into our living habits.

Food is the first place we learn self-regulation. We learn to stop eating when we are full, to choose healthy options, to slow down in the face of "goodies," and to learn how to treat ourselves and respect our bodies. Think about how much and how often we eat at the behest of others: We eat because they say it is time to eat, we eat what they want us to eat, we eat to please them, we eat as much as they want us to eat, or we struggle with food because we want to look a certain way for others. Eating is clearly a behavior that is about our bodies, and our minds, and yet so much of the time we do it in the service of others, and most troublesome, we find it difficult to walk away from a half-full plate of food even when we are done.

Food is our first lesson in self-regulation, and all of our other self-regulation lessons stem from our relationship with food and our ability to adjust it.

LIFE'S OTHER PLATES

Our eating patterns tend to mirror our behavior in other areas of our lives, such as love, work, and money. We are told to blindly follow rules when it comes to food, such as:

- Eat what is on your plate.

- Eat to please.

- Even if other people give you what you don't want, finish it up.

- Even if you initially choose badly or put too much on your plate, tough luck—finish up.

Now what if we substituted eat with love, money, and work. What if we said:

- Love the way others want you to love.

- Spend to please others.

- Stick it out even if it's not working, even if you initially didn't choose well.

That doesn't feel good, does it? Few of us are genuinely socialized to listen to ourselves, which is an elegant balance of analyzing the data, integrating it, and then listening. It also means hearing what our stakeholders have to say but then still honoring ourselves. We have to face down the fear, too. Keep in mind that fear is often what knits tribes of stakeholders together, and we erroneously believe that if one person does what feels right, then anarchy may break out. We have been so programmed to march to the call of others, to listen to others, that not only do we not know how to eat, but we are also losing sight of how to live.

Ultimately when you take responsibility and ownership, whether at the dinner table, in the bedroom, or at work, you are taking a risk. It is a risk because if you fail, it's "your fault." I am always amazed at how awful a feeling it is for people, even when they trust their guts, to have to take responsibility.

Let's draw a specific parallel here. Just like you did in chapter 8, I want you to think about some of the reasons why you eat:

- To avoid bad feelings

- To give yourself a reward

- To fill the emptiness
- To manage frustration
- Loneliness
- Anger
- Fear
- Boredom
- Because the world tells you to eat

Now, think about some of the reasons you have been (or perhaps currently are) in a bad relationship. Are you finding any similarities?

- To avoid being alone
- To give yourself a reward from the outside
- To fill an emptiness
- To manage loneliness
- Because you are afraid to be alone
- Boredom
- Because the world tells you to

Are those also the reasons you may spend money the way you do? Or stay in a job you don't like?

It is a house of cards. By denying our spider senses, we can maintain the illusion. It's why we often take stock and find ourselves at an unhealthy weight and unhappy in many other things. Remember: Fear, stakeholders, and golden rules are loud. And spider senses do not tend to operate in just one area. Once you unleash them and listen to them, you may start shifting your role in a relationship after you lose weight, or you may start questioning your job, or you may start approaching many other things in your life differently. Once you stop living blindly in one province, you will stop living blindly in all of them. Spider senses don't know walls.

In the next few chapters, we are going to take the central tenets of this book—our spider senses, our stakeholders, our fears, and our golden rules—and apply them to gatekeeping and walking away in our relationships, our jobs, and our lives in general. You will start to see that your compulsion to blindly finish everything on your plate may in fact be a glimpse into why you are sticking out a broken relationship, a broken job, and a broken life. Once you are courageous enough to walk away from that second helping, you may become strong enough to walk away from other things, too. Believe it or not, that clean plate may be about more than just your weight.

The next few chapters examine how society wants us to fit a certain role, and this book is about breaking out of that role and those scripts. I don't think the fact that we find ourselves in an epidemic of obesity is very surprising; after all, our society as a whole is invested in everyone following a party line, whether it's eating, loving, spending, working, or living. You can break your habits, but first it requires that you be willing to break with society and listen to yourself.

CHAPTER 13

Love and Relationships: When Do You Hold and When Do You Fold?

In art as in love, instinct is enough.

—Anatole France

A popular relationship weight-loss myth in our culture sounds like this: "Oh look, she lost the weight and got a divorce, and now that she's skinny, she is trading up / getting rid of him / thinks she is better than him." This is a childish take on a complex situation. Making the commitment to lose weight and successfully achieving that goal means taking on lots of changes, both large and small. It means valuing oneself enough to actually become healthier; it means saying no to unhealthy options; it means making time for exercise. And all of this means less time for something (or someone) else. Mounting a successful weight-loss effort means learning to advocate for yourself. It means listening to yourself.

And that is bound to segue into the rest of life. Learning to walk away from a second helping may very well translate into clearer communication within relationships and standing up for yourself. That could result in a stronger, healthier relationship, or it could result in needing to walk away from something that is no longer nourishing. By learning to listen to your spider senses—knowing when you are full, and knowing when to walk away from the plate—you start learning to trust your spider senses in all areas of your relationships. You may trust your spider senses and ask for something you need, or address something that makes you uncomfortable, rather than numbing those feelings.

The pattern of losing weight and ending relationships is often simplified into a scenario where the person who lost weight now "looks good" and is "on the prowl." The more likely scenario is that sustained and healthy weight loss may require the person to learn to take care of him- or herself, and the day-after-day process of feeding a body with healthy food, making better choices, and advocating for oneself at the table may translate into greater advocacy in a relationship, and a better ability to communicate needs and recognize wants. It is also likely that a successful weight-loss process, characterized by listening to spider senses, opens up those spider senses everywhere in the person's life, including his or her relationships.

Like food, relationships are a primitive place. Many of our lessons were learned early on by watching our parents and taking cues from the world around us. We are in many ways wired to make the same mistakes over and over again, and much of this is due to our inability to heed our spider senses. Think about most of the bad relationships you have had: You can almost trace back to the moment in time when you knew it was wrong, but the voices around you, the golden rules, and the fears within you told you to "stick it out."

Relationships also become a tricky balancing act. They require treading that fine line of spider senses and good sense in order to make the right decision. Ironically, most people enter marriage far more frivolously than a mortgage—at least a mortgage has a finite end—and the legal and financial entanglements of a marriage reach far more deeply. At the end of the day the main lesson we are taught about relationships is that the only successful way for a marriage to end is if one of the parties dies—"'til death do us part." If someone leaves voluntarily, then it gets chalked up to failure. People get congratulated on the longevity of their relationships, but rarely are they asked, "Has it been a happy twenty years?" Why is divorce deemed a failure rather than simply an end?

By and large when we eat badly, we are treating ourselves badly. Many times I have watched someone eat an excessive meal in the name of "treating" themselves. The fact is, many people do not know how to treat themselves and are experts at putting themselves down. In fact, if most of us were in a relationship with ourselves, we should break up with us, given how badly we treat ourselves. So if we are treating ourselves badly through food, it makes sense to stay in a relationship that is not working. Why would we value ourselves in that space either?

The fact is, many people do not know how to treat themselves and are experts at putting themselves down. In fact, if most of us were in a relationship with ourselves, we should break up with us, given how badly we treat ourselves.

PRESERVE AT ALL COSTS?

We are caught in a cult of "preserve the relationship" at any cost. What is unfortunate is that so many people are poor gate-keepers at the time they choose a life partner. Maybe they are young, or still haven't figured out who they are and what they want. Many times we choose partners, particularly those we choose earlier in life, on the basis of what we know, and that is generally the party line fed to us by our families and our communities. We tend to choose people who look like us, work like us, are educated like us, and who make "good prospects." Good prospects are typically defined by society—money, ambition, vocation, and demographic characteristics. Rarely does authenticity climb too high on that list. People will look askance at the woman committed to the genuine, authentic (albeit money-less) artist, but they will often jump into reveries of celebration for those who may choose an unkind (albeit wealthy) financier. Our spider senses can be all but silenced in the relationship realm when we are faced with our stakeholders. So while we might make a bad choice, we're often forced into that feeling of being stuck with it. We all make bad choices; we shouldn't have to pay for them forever.

STAKEHOLDERS AND LOVE

Even more than at the dinner table, stakeholders exert an incredibly powerful influence on us in relationships. They set the tone for us early on for what we should expect, and we learn from watching their relationships. They voice approval and disapproval, so not only can they significantly impact gatekeeping, but they are also critical in keeping us in unhealthy relationships even after our spider senses do kick in. Even when our spider senses are screaming *Get out,* our stakeholders are saying *Stay in.*

I talked to dozens of people about their dating lives, courtships, relationships, marriages, and divorces in preparing this book. One theme that was surprisingly common was ambivalence at the altar, or even earlier in the relationship. Many of these people basically shared that they knew, at the spider-sense level, that it was not the right fit, but they assumed that with time, it would grow to be right. In almost all cases that person "looked good on paper": He or she had the right job, the right family, and it was the right time to get hitched. Some of these marriages and relationships are still intact, but some have ended.

GATEKEEPING AND LOVE

Timing is everything, they say. In life, opportunities are often presented to us at times when we cannot avail ourselves of them. For example, children make a move for a promising new job more difficult; you meet a wonderful potential partner but are already in a relationship. The same thing happens with food: We eat lunch and then get to work and a lunch buffet is set out; the big dinner out falls on the day we feel sick; we start a healthier food regimen and the new administrative assistant brings donuts in every morning. Gatekeeping and spider senses are critical in navigating the tricky waters of timing and opportunities.

Obviously when we meet that right person at the right time, that's a good thing. Often such people reflect on their good luck or the fact that they constructed the opportunity. For example, they were actively dating, attending social functions, or going to online dating sites. Spider senses operate to tell us this is the right person, and gatekeeping operates for us to let them in—and it works. Keep in mind, too, that if you are listening to your spider senses, then you are likely taking care of yourself in other areas of your life (e.g., eating well, exercising), and are more willing to put yourself out in the world. Many people who struggle with weight or body-image issues will report that they don't feel ready to put themselves out there. Often when working with a client who is struggling with both weight and relationship issues, we focus on unearthing those spider senses and reminding her to take care of herself, so that she will be positioned to engage in some good relationship gatekeeping.

Spider senses become essential when you face bad timing and the right person. This can become a morally sticky issue. Can a married person leave a shaky marriage because they find a better partner? What about someone who is engaged? Just a boyfriend? Doesn't that mean every relationship is hanging in a state of suspended animation, waiting for a "better" person to poach one of the partners away? I would argue no. In a committed, connected, and authentic relationship, the parties are invested in each other, the connection is powerful, both are growing and secure, and even if a bevy of beauties or other engaging new opportunities are paraded in front of either person, the investment in the relationship and the authentic connection implies that such "temptations" will not result in either of them running away.

By and large, I see the darker relationship failures such as infidelity occur when there is a certain lack of authenticity operating, such as relationships glued together by obligation, stakeholders, fears, or golden rules. And don't get me wrong—those glues are mighty strong. But they are also false, and as a result the behavior of the parties within the relationship starts drifting to an inauthentic place, because the people in the relationship are unable to walk away from a dirty plate. It's a bit like the person who keeps eating even though he is full because he doesn't want to deal with the other things that need to be managed in his life.

Where it gets tricky is when the marriage or relationship is not working, and the person is fighting to keep it intact, throwing bad money after good, staying at the table, cleaning the plate. It is at this nexus that we see infidelity, dubious conduct on the Internet, and a fantasy life that starts to encroach on real life. It takes courage to sift through the wreckage, to see if it can be fixed, have the painful but necessary conversations, but then walk away when it is broken, just like you'd walk away from a plate that still has some food on it when you are full.

Ask anyone who has walked away, and they'll tell you that divorce or a breakup of a long-term relationship was one of the most difficult decisions they ever had to make. But there are times when the person in that broken relationship realizes that they would be healthier out of that partnership. Obviously, the best course of action is when the married person works with his or her partner to either remediate the relationship or disassemble it. At such times, spider senses become critical, and it can be tricky business with the overpowering din of stakeholders, the intoxicating mythologies of fairy tales that reinforce people for sticking it out, and the fear of being alone and leaving the safe, known (yet broken) place for the unknown.

It comes back to what we already discussed about positive and negative reinforcement. Staying in a relationship may work from the position of negative *reinforcement,* because by staying or by getting into a relationship, whether you want it or not, you get other people off your back. So when you stick around or you get into a relationship, it's easier than dealing with the criticism and disillusionment and fears. Many people I have talked to have said, "I got a boyfriend to shut my mother up. . . ."

Here's a situation in which people get into hot water in the first place: The time is right, your friends are all getting married or are in relationships, you finally have the right job and now want the right partner, your biological clock is ticking, and so you take the most reasonable option that presents itself at that time. Many people have ignored their spider senses and made the classical gatekeeping error, thinking, "If I don't marry this one, another one might never come along." Fear feeds into the bad pick: fear about being alone, fear about missing the boat, fear of failing to please stakeholders, or fear of failing to meet a societal script.

It's easy to walk away from the wrong person at the wrong time. If it's not the right time, you are not noticing anyone. And if you meet someone who is clearly not a good fit in any way, it's even easier to say good-bye.

Interestingly, most people use relationship counseling (marriage counseling, couples counseling, etc.) at the wrong time. Typically people turn to a counselor once the whole system starts falling apart, and by then it is often too late. My professional advice is to seek out the services of a licensed mental health practitioner with expertise in relationship counseling *before* you sign on the dotted line or make a more permanent commitment. It is a chance to use an important data source at the time of gatekeeping and get training in communication, listening, support, and opening up about vulnerabilities within your relationship. Instead of using counseling as a place of dismantling, it is actually a wonderful place to gatekeep and strengthen your relationship at the front end.

FEAR AND LOVE

There is a song lyric from a popular song that goes something like "Fear is the heart of love." It's sad and cynical, but unfortunately, we have allowed it to become true. I see more fear in relationships than in any other arena in which I work—fear of getting hurt, fear of being rejected, fear of being alone, fear of dying, fear of change, fear of never having a child, fear of what others will think, fear of letting down your family, or fear of letting down your children.

Fear is the most powerful adhesive we have. Fear unites, because if two people are afraid, then even as the authentic ties that may have once bound them disappear, the fear ties are as sticky as a spider's web. I am amazed at how many relationships are cemented by fear rather than connection. Interestingly, with many people I know who struggle with food and walking away, one of the fears is "When will I get to eat again?" So we often eat more than we should in fear of not having enough. Perhaps we stay in relationships longer than we should for a similar reason—the fear of not having enough love, attention, or affiliation.

Fear is the most powerful adhesive we have. Fear unites, because if two people are afraid, then even as the authentic ties that may have once bound them disappear, the fear ties are as sticky as a spider's web.

We have talked about fear and how it fools with spider senses. The fears are not rational; the most classical fears all emanate from the relationship space. Freud wisely said about love: "We are never so defenseless against suffering as when we love." And these fears are fires that get their oxygen from our stakeholders, who fill us with fears of shame or reinforce our existing fears and keep the fire going. And because so many people around us are living in relationships that may need to be dismantled, or at least reconfigured, you can find yourself in a tribe where everyone has drunk the Kool-Aid and no one is heeding their spider senses.

I find it fascinating that 54 percent of Americans will eat until their plates are empty; it's a similar statistic for the divorce rate in the United States. Maybe the dirty-platers are the ones who are leaving relationships? When I look at the people I have talked to who have taken bold stances in their relationships and walked away, they noticed that the stakeholders who often most distanced themselves from their situation were those who were in questionable relationships. Simply the action of that person walking away was a bit more of a wake-up call than their stakeholders were able to tolerate. So instead of facing what may have been going on in their own lives, they did what most relationship ostriches do: They stuck their heads in the sand.

The classic fear is, "If I communicate my needs and he doesn't like it, he will leave me." If he would leave you for communicating your needs, what kind of life is that setting up for you? If your partner cannot hear your dreams, your hopes, your needs, your wants, and your concerns, and would leave if you voiced them, why would you want to keep that relationship? This is most likely a tone that is set early in the relationship.

I recently spoke with a woman who was going through a divorce after fourteen years of marriage. Her husband was a wealthy man with a successful medical practice. They had two children. When they initially came together she had a successful career, and he encouraged her to leave it. He said he would take care of her, and they were going to have kids, so why work? She told me about the detritus of their relationship: infidelities, strippers, sex workers, and insults. And the very guy who had encouraged her to leave her career was now criticizing her for spending but not earning. She talked about how narcissistic he was (and he was!), always putting his needs above the needs of everyone else.

I then asked her if this was really a change, or if he'd been like that when she met him. She confessed that he had always been like that. But the game was different fifteen years ago when they were courting. He was considered a "good catch." Her friends were getting married, she wanted kids, he was rich, he said he would take care of her, and so the narcissism seemed like a nagging fly—even though she did acknowledge that it hadn't sat well with her at the time (spider senses). She went ahead and assumed it would "just work itself out." It didn't. It rarely does.

The person you meet is who they have always been at a fundamental and core level. He didn't change, but being in the presence of his entitlement for so long wore on her. She never tried to talk to him about her concerns early on; after all, her mother had told her how lucky she was to have him, her married friends enjoyed spending time with them, and even as her spider senses kept telling her to get out, she fought to stay in until she was faced with the mountain of evidence that he had been repeatedly having sexual relationships outside of the marriage. It was consistent with his behavior from day one. If she had communicated her needs early on and he left her, wouldn't she have been better off?

THE RELATIONSHIP BAIT AND SWITCH

This is a situation where gatekeeping, stakeholders, and fairy tales often come together in a dreadful collision that can set the tone for long-term dishonest and inauthentic relationships. You know about the bait and switch—for example, you go to a car dealership advertising the make and model of a car you want for $12,000, just at the top of your budget. But when you get there, you find out the car lacks features you thought it would have, and by the time the correct car is offered to you, it now costs $5,000 more. The bait was the low price that got you into the dealership, and then the salesperson got you to pay the higher price because you were hooked and in the mindset of wanting to buy a car. Such a maneuver can leave you feeling tricked.

Relationships are the same. Often when we meet new people, they get the "best" version of us—a well-put-together, great-conversationalist, upbeat version. Many times in life, we hit periods when we want to be in a relationship; we think it's time to get married, our parents are pressuring us, we are afraid to be alone, we want someone to take trips with. At those times, if we find a potential partner in whom we may be interested, we might say and do things that are not really what we are all about. In essence, we defy our spider senses. For example, we may say we want kids when we don't, or that we love football when we don't, or that we like certain foods that we don't. We often create a different version of ourselves to first bait and then hook the other person, and once we feel secure in the relationship, we come clean and the baby-loving, football-loving, carnivore you presented yourself to be turns out to be someone quite different. Or worse, you hold back on communicating needs or wants for fear of losing the person and then find yourself years into a relationship where you still cannot communicate about what you need or want. Many times we do the bait and switch for reasons of fear, fantasy, or pressure from the outside world. Word to the wise: Let the used-car dealers keep the bait and switch; relationships are no place for denying spider senses and turning yourself into someone you're not. It's simply not sustainable.

THE GOLDEN RULES AND LOVE

Cinderella worked hard, was obedient, found mice to make her clothes, played hard-to-get, lost a shoe, found a prince, and lived happily ever after. We were raised on this nonsense, girls in particular—the stuff that reinforced gender roles, assured us we would be rescued and that relationships were safe.

We also learned the golden rules about listening to our parents, not wasting stuff, and honoring vows (even if they were made from an uninformed space). What's interesting to me is that if a person were in a job that did not pay well, was going nowhere, and was causing distress, and then that person found a new job that paid better, we would not criticize him or her for making that shift. If a person is in a relationship or marriage that is not fulfilling or healthy, going nowhere, causing distress, and that person found an alternative mate who treated her better and left, many would call her a selfish bitch for making that shift.

Weddings and the surplus meaning of relationships can definitely scramble spider senses. What is it about vows made in a white dress that are so much more compelling than other sorts of promises? I am a huge proponent of renewable vows that require revisiting, re-crafting, and reconsidering every five years. I am also a serious supporter of vows to oneself—because if you can't adhere to your promises to yourself, are you really going to be able to love, honor, and cherish another? This requires growth rather than complacence or blind allegiance, and it requires the parties to stay in touch with their spider senses.

The good thing about staying in touch with spider senses within a relationship is that it forces you to communicate with your partner, honor yourself, and take care of yourself. If there is one huge risk for people in relationships, it's that they outsource their needs. So much of our relationship fantasy in this culture centers around being rescued. In outsourcing our needs and waiting to be rescued, the fairy tales of youth start looming large, and any time we outsource, our spider senses lose their edge. Spider senses make you better in a relationship from the outset, because instead of letting sleeping dogs lie, you actually address problems as they arise because things don't feel right. Instead of letting a situation fester to the point of no return, you take it on at the time and insert growth rather than disease into a relationship. However, communicating clearly means facing fears, and that is a tough pill for people to swallow.

BUT ISN'T IT ALL ABOUT THE WEDDING?

Ah, the wedding . . . contributor to gatekeeping errors on the biggest decision you can make in a life. The wedding is the ultimate scrambler of our good judgment and our spider senses, and it impairs our gatekeeping, big-time. I love love—everyone loves love, and everyone loves a party. I don't think a lifelong legal commitment should be made just for the sake of having a party. The wedding is the best example of a gatekeeping mistake with permanent ramifications. Let's face it, love in the beginning (four to eighteen months into a relationship, depending on the couple) is all good; it's all dopamine. Every time you see this person, it's like doing a line of cocaine or eating fudge—the same brain areas light up. You are bright, shiny, beautiful, and it's wonderful. It makes sense that you would want to celebrate it with your friends. It could be the ultimate gatekeeping error. Don't legally link yourself to someone just so you can have a big party, look pretty, and have your friends celebrate with you.

Remember, too, sometimes one thing leads to another and you get swept up in saying yes to a proposal, and yes to getting married, when you really knew on your second date with this person that this was a bad fit, and that you should have walked away. It gets more and more difficult to get up and walk away once the hall is booked, the dress is purchased, and the invites are in the mail, so you have to gatekeep early and tap into your spider senses, because once the food is on the plate, or the wedding train has left the station, canceling is much more difficult. Basically, don't put the cookies on the plate, and if you don't like him, don't go on the second date.

The problem with weddings is that they are something we are socialized to dream about, a cultural archetype. Celebrating falling in love is fabulous. It is that most human and lush of experiences. Marriage, however, is legally binding, and it places a regulatory and sometimes religious imprimatur on a relationship. It sets up tax benefits, a way to share assets, and simplifies probate. It's like establishing an LLC or some other corporate structure: It provides protection. Did you throw a formal party the day you signed your car loan? Did you throw a party when you closed on your home? Was your drunken uncle in the room when you went in to sign paperwork that legally bound you to a home?

In most cases, people cannot make a lifelong commitment after a month, but they can be in love after a month. The hard work of really mulling over the ramifications of marriage is tough, and such a decision should take place with reason, advisement, and focus. People should consult experts before getting married, and always, always return to their spider senses. But in the rush to have a party, all that irritating stuff gets swept aside. I am astonished at the number of people who have confessed that they knew on their wedding day, from a spider-sense-y place, that it didn't feel right. But in the mad dash to avoid disappointing their parents and caterers, the fear of being alone, and missing out on the fairytale wedding, mistakes get made.

The wedding is clearly governed by a social order. It's as though without a legal contract we cannot celebrate love, and it speaks to how much our thinking about relationships is colored by the world in which we live.

BAD MONEY AFTER GOOD—BUT LOVE IS NOT MONEY

As Americans, we tend to view relationships like money or an expensive meal, and lots of people will often resist leaving a long-term relationship, saying, "I invested so much time into it; how can I leave?" A relationship is not a bank account or a steak dinner. Yes, you may have accumulated assets and such, but it was simply the process of your life. Stakeholders, fears, and golden rules about how to allocate assets all squirm in the face of someone trying to leave a long relationship, as they may view those twenty years as wasted. I argue the contrary. Such a relationship was a beautiful and important part of your life, and that vision of it can remain if you don't stick it out to the point where it gets rancorous.

Relationships, like all human experiences, are transient; they change every day and are meant to be enjoyed in the present. When I hear people say you need to "work" at a relationship, what that often really means is just seeing through the day-to-day: listening to another person, listening to yourself, not getting stuck on hurts from the past, and not getting lost in what might come. To be in a relationship with someone you respect, care about, and value is a gift, and when you take that in the day-to-day, you honor yourself and your partner each day. Eating is no different in that you can honor yourself at each meal. So much time in relationships is spent hashing the past and arguing about things that haven't yet happened. A relationship cannot be "hoarded," just like a meal cannot be prolonged by taking home the leftovers.

Some relationships may last twenty minutes, some twenty weeks, some twenty years, and some until you die. There is no prize at the end for sticking it out. The length of a relationship is not an indicator of its success, and perhaps the real measure of success, just like at the table, is the ability to listen to yourself, get the most out of it, and, in some cases, walk away before the world thinks you should.

Human relationships are not just with a spouse or intimate partner—relationships are with family members, children, friends, and colleagues. And all of the rules above apply. You don't have to stick out any relationship because you feel obligated. You can fix it or you can walk away from it. You can also learn to consume it differently. But retaining the status quo because of fear, because of golden rules that you didn't write, is like selling yourself down the river. Life is short, and our social connections are one of

If you are going to go to the trouble of choosing healthy food for your plate, shouldn't you also choose healthy people for your life?

the most important things in our world, so shouldn't they be healthy? If you are going to go to the trouble of choosing healthy food for your plate, shouldn't you also choose healthy people for your life? I am confident that as you start making healthier choices at the table, you will make healthier choices in people as well.

Few books or experts advocate marital dismantling; we are, in fact, quite obsessed as a culture with keeping them together. Unfortunately, we do not give people in our culture the skills they need to gatekeep and construct good relationships, but we do ask them to keep these broken structures together. I have a problem with not teaching those skills and then demanding that people live with their errors indefinitely and make them work.

RELATIONSHIPS AND THE "CLOUD"

Even though we don't really "lose" our history when a relationship or marriage ends, we do lose our shared custodian of those memories. He may remember the color of the car you rented on your honeymoon; you remember the flavor of the wedding cake. Works out nicely—you don't have to remember all the details because the other person may hold on to different stuff than you. Thus, the end of the relationship means that the shared historian isn't so close anymore and neither are those memories and factoids. It goes back to the old adage "two heads are better than one." Unfortunately, this sharing of the memory "load" can lead us to hold on to broken relationships. A committed relationship is like the "cloud." It's like sharing information on a network rather than on just one hard drive, and it can be a more efficient use of space. But, efficiency can sometimes make us lazy.

BUT WHAT ABOUT THE KIDS?

Kids are the ultimate stakeholders, and when we split from a spouse or partner, everyone always wonders, "What about the kids?"

I will acknowledge, and this is supported by research, that divorce is hard on children. When I work with patients whose parents are divorced, they will admit that it was a turning point in their lives. My twelve-year-old daughter, when asked to write an essay about a difficult experience, wrote about our divorce.

That said, there is also significant harm that can come from growing up in a home characterized by discord. Ideally, we make good gatekeeping choices before having kids, but often we don't. And frankly, sometimes we do, even if the marriage ends. My ex-husband is a fantastic father, and while he and I didn't make it, I am tremendously grateful he is their father. I am a firm believer that if you plan on marrying someone and having kids, you should choose a person who will be a good parent. Odds are fifty-fifty or so that the marriage may end, but they are 100 percent that the person will always be the child's parent. Choose wisely for the sake of the child who didn't have a say in the matter. Sexy rich guy may seem like an alluring partner, but what happens when it's time for diapers and discipline?

"Sticking it out for the kids" is another example of outsourcing: You get to play martyr, and yet your children are raised in a climate of disconnection that is inauthentic. In the long run, window dressing teaches a set of lessons that may be more destructive than managing the rupture of a family. That said, I know my daughters will always struggle with our divorce, just as they may have struggled with an unhappy home if we had stuck it out. Choose your misery. My work as a mother then becomes remaining respectful of their father, working on our friendship, and retaining my spider senses so I can guide my children well.

In order to stay in a relationship that does not work, you need to silence parts of yourself. Sadly, you are likely silencing your spider senses. By silencing your spider senses, you may stay in a broken relationship. Over time, you are reinforced for shutting down those spider senses: Everyone is happy you stuck it out, you don't have to face your fears, and you are heeding the golden rule of "Winners don't quit." But to do so, you had to silence yourself, and this can have damaging consequences. In talking to people in relationships that were pretty awful, I have noticed that they silenced—and subsequently lost—themselves over time because if they hadn't, the relationship could not have continued. In the end, they were not feeling self-congratulatory, but rather bitter and resentful.

THE WHY

When relationships have outlived their shelf life, people often realize that at some level, they are sticking it out because they once thought in the light of their divine love that the other person would change. Sorry for breaking the poetic hope here, but that doesn't happen. People are like rubber bands: They may be able to stretch from time to time and do some amazing things, but in general they are who they are. If manipulation and machinations on your side get them to behave the way you want, I will set my clock on the fact that they will return to their previous way of behaving, or they will just keep faking it. To be in a relationship with someone who is not really there doesn't make sense. People who aren't cooperating can often feel like a project to us, like something for us to rescue or fix. Rescuing is the province of firefighters and fairy tales, but it's not real life. The stance of sticking it out in hopes of redemption is an old story and one that has wasted many lives. It's a passive strategy, and one that does not work in life, or at the table.

Culture is also a cop-out to me. I recognize this because I lived it. Nice Indian girls don't get divorced. I was even sold a bill of goods that if the eldest daughter does not get married, then, according to the rules of reincarnation, the father will have worse prospects in the next life. Talk about stakeholder pressure! I am amazed at the relativism we use when understanding a construct such as culture. Rules are modified within various cultures as technology and society progresses. For example, people in remote villages learn to use cell phones, but these same villagers will still employ ancient and cruel punishments on girls who won't get married or who leave their marriages. The idea that one has to get married and that one has to stay married in the name of culture is an outsourcing rather than a taking of responsibility for one's authentic life. I know that in Indian culture, in addition to not walking away from relationships, you also don't leave food behind on your plate. This left me fat and unhappy. It may be harder to make certain changes when they are at odds with cultural demands, but that doesn't mean they can't be made. I am tired of ancient and outmoded cultural rules holding people back from fulfilled lives.

The bottom line: It's okay to walk away. Nothing bad will happen. Weigh your options, but don't think time will fix an ailing marriage. The fairy tales about sticking it out, the conventional wisdom about persisting, and the ways that stakeholders and fears hurt both our gatekeeping and our spider senses requires courage and facing down old scripts.

It's also okay to use data for guidance in how we conduct ourselves in relationships. Obviously, we *do* care what other people think about our partner, and we may want advice on things like having children, getting a divorce, or sticking it out. As Daniel Gilbert brilliantly opines in *Stumbling on Happiness,* talk to people who are where you want to be. Want to walk away? Talk to someone who has walked away. But always take all that data and bring it home to your spider senses. Let it breathe, and then you can take on your decisions using both data and your own intuition.

THE NOW

The exercise here is tougher, because as a reader of this book, you may be any number of things: happily in a committed relationship, unhappily in a committed relationship, happily single, or unhappily single. So I would like to give each of these four groups some tasks to take on to ensure that spider senses are being honored in their relationships.

Happy in Your Relationship

This is like a garden that is in bloom, and you always want it to stay that way. Then cultivate it:

- Ensure that you regularly, yet honestly, share gratitude and positive thoughts and feelings with your partner. We are good at pointing out the things our partners do wrong; take the time to show him/her that you notice the good stuff.

- Use "I feel" statements so you can express feelings and take ownership of them.

- Make time for the relationship. Just like a garden, you have to weed and water a relationship, and doing that when things are good may give you the tools to manage things during rough patches.

- Touch base—practice relationship mindfulness, and pay attention. Just like you shouldn't eat mindlessly, you shouldn't relate mindlessly, either.

- Reflect on how you honor your spider senses in your relationship and ensure that it's occurring in other areas as well.

Unhappy in Your Relationship

This is a tough one. This book isn't going to be a palliative for a broken relationship or marriage. If you and your partner are experiencing significant relationship distress, be sure to get counseling with a licensed mental health practitioner. Here are some questions to ask yourself now:

- What are your spider senses telling you about this relationship?
- What do you wish was different?
- What would you keep the same?
- What are you afraid would happen if you stayed together?
- What are you afraid would happen if you parted ways?
- What were you told about relationships when you were a child?
- What do your stakeholders want (especially your heavy stakeholders)?
- What is the nature of your communication with your partner (indifferent, argumentative, angry, insulting)?
- What did your spider senses tell you at the time of gatekeeping (when you got together)?

These are great questions for you to figure out for yourself, and may prepare you to start having conversations with each other and with a professional as well.

Happy and Single

It's a nice place to be, and this is often a wonderful time to really shore up your spider senses, take ownership of your mental and physical health, and enjoy the many other relationships in your life.

Reflect on what you were taught about relationships while growing up, and how that has impacted your decision to not be in a committed relationship right now.

Consider how you might react if you did meet someone interesting. Reflect on how fears, golden rules, and stakeholders would factor into your thinking and gatekeeping. You may be committed to being relationship-free for a lifetime; if that's congruent with what you want, then honor that, but by reflecting on these themes now, if things should someday shift for you, you may be in a better position to gatekeep down the road.

Unhappy and Single

Dating in a modern age is no small task. But with the lessons from this book, you are in a great position to start honoring your spider senses, meeting people, and doing some solid gatekeeping. Just like with diet and exercise, you already know what a healthy relationship looks like. And you probably know about online dating, getting yourself out there, and trying to meet people. This book is not a how-to book on dating. It will, however, give you the most powerful dating tip of all: honoring your voice so you can put a version of you that honors yourself out there into the world, and subsequently attract a partner who does the same. In addition, by doing this you will value you, and in your quest, while still single, enjoy the wonder that is you. Ask yourself the following questions:

- What are your fears about getting into a relationship?
- What are your fears about being alone?
- What do your stakeholders want for you?
- What are the golden rules and scripts that you take into a new relationship?
- What are your hopes about what a relationship will bring into your life?
- What are your fears about getting into a relationship?

"GREAT ON-PAPER" EXERCISE

Be very careful that you don't turn dating into an employment application. Think about what you really want. Listen, ladies—if wealth is actually important to you, at a spider-sense level, then own it, but also own everything that may imply. Does it cut to the core of a fear about your inability to take care of yourself? Of what your family wants for you? List the traits you think your stakeholders want you to find in a partner; then list the traits that you want in a partner. Look at the disconnects, because those disconnects may also be holding you back.

SELF-NURTURANCE

This exercise is important for everyone, but particularly for those who are either unhappily partnered or unpartnered. Often it is those who are in unhappy relational spaces who do not take good care of themselves—eating poorly, not doing nice things for themselves, not exercising, and so on. I have my patients make a list of daily nurturances (things that aren't very time-consuming that could be done any day, or every day), such as taking a bath or taking a walk. I also have them record weekly nurturances—things that may take a little more time or money, such as a manicure, massage, or going to a basketball game with friends. Schedule some of the weekly ones and start engaging in the daily ones. Taking care of yourself will help you put yourself out there in a more bold and self-loving manner.

Finally, all of these exercises are relevant to all relationships in your life—if you have a great relationship with Mom, use some of the "happy relationship" tips to cultivate that. If you are estranged from your sister, use some of the "unhappy relationship" tips there. If you wish you had more friends, use some of those "unhappy single" tips.

PROMISE OF ONE: LOVE AND RELATIONSHIPS

Use the Promise of One to nurture the relationship you are in, nurture yourself, or nurture the other relationships in your life. Once a day, find a way to connect with a partner, connect with yourself, connect with loved ones, express gratitude. In this case, the Promise of One will allow you to take a moment every day and nurture the garden of people in your world, which will result in growth and health for you and others.

CHECK-IN: LOVE

No matter where you are in life—single, married, in love, separated, or separating—think about love and relationships and what love should look like to you. What elements of love do you love? Reflect on your current situation, and remain mindful of whether you are relying on a script to dictate what love looks like, or actually listening to your spider senses and allowing it to unfold organically and naturally. Why write the ending ahead of time?

CHAPTER 14

Full from Your Job?
Follow Your Dream

You have a right to experiment with your life. You will make mistakes. And they are right too. . . . I think we have a right to change course. But society is the one that keeps demanding that we fit in and not disturb things.

—Anaïs Nin

I don't think weight prevents us from being functioning professionals, but I think it might hold us back from chasing our dreams. Maintaining the status quo in how we eat can actually translate into maintaining the status quo in how we work and live. That's why it's important to understand that trusting our gut and spider senses can have major ramifications for work. Many times sticking out an unsatisfying job is no different than maintaining an unhealthy weight or unhealthy relationship—with similar patterns of numbly going through the day-to-day routine, never questioning, blindly consuming what is in front of you, being concerned with the input of stakeholders, and making bad choices from a place of fear. If you don't think you can leave food on your plate, how could you ever envision leaving a job you've had for fifteen years? We *are* allowed to change course, despite the pressures of society that demand otherwise.

If your spider senses tell you that your current job is terrible and going nowhere and you don't have another job, the hope is that you will try to secure other employment, perhaps even temporary, so you can walk away from a bad situation and still address your responsibilities. Work and finances raise numerous issues around responsibility, and one of the basic tenets of this book is that by being honest and listening to yourself, you are more likely to take responsibility. Society takes an interesting stance here: We view people, particularly men, as providers, and as long as you are bringing in the money and paying your bills, you are being responsible. Even if you are in a dissatisfying job that leaves you empty at the end of the day. We probably spend more waking hours working than doing anything else; thus, lack of satisfaction there can really take a toll.

I had the opportunity in my life to test out my spider senses in a job. When I finished my graduate work I was in a postdoctoral position, which over time became unfulfilling, with little opportunity for growth. It was in an impressive setting, working with prestigious people, but over time I saw that it would go nowhere and not give me the autonomy I desperately wanted. My spider senses said *Jump!* Stakeholders weighed in about the issues involved in leaving such a prestigious place. I knew my supervisor was not going to be pleased, and I was afraid no one else would hire me—or that it would be worse elsewhere. While I stayed in the job, I noticed that other things in my life were also not going well— the longer I was in that job, the more (and worse) I ate. I was denying my spider senses by going to work each day, so of course they would stop working in my eating habits as well. Nonetheless, I heeded my spider senses, applied for the professorship I am still in today, and got it.

One of the hard things about leaving that first job was my belief that if I stuck it out, I might advance within a more prestigious institution, or other more "exciting" things would come my way if I stayed. But my gut and the data I had accumulated up to that point did not support this likelihood. I left and found a new job that has its own issues (like every job does), but it has been gratifying in many ways, and it has allowed me to develop as a scholar and a teacher, which is what I wanted. Interestingly, about ten years later, I ran into one of my coworkers from that previous job. She and some others had entered the job at the same time I did. I was fascinated to learn that neither she nor anyone else in the job had developed the kinds of opportunities I had assumed we would all gain by sticking it out there. It would have been a dead end, which confirmed for me that my spider senses had been dead-on a decade earlier. This revelation made me trust my spider senses even more.

HONORING YOUR DREAMS AND PAYING THE BILLS

It is critical to know what you want in a job—not just what you will do, but the characteristics of the job. Some people love freedom and are willing to take work home, or even sacrifice salary to have more flexibility; some people like having boundaries and knowing that when they clock out at the end of day, they're done. Some people welcome travel; others abhor it. Some people want balance, while others don't mind eighteen-hour days. You are the only one who knows you—and as with relationships, there has to be compromise. Some jobs may require eighteen-hour days at one point in the year, but not others. Think about rhythms that matter to you. At the end of this chapter I'm going to provide you with a way to honestly assess what your present job offers, and what you want.

Just like with food and relationships, work is about a position of compromise. We have to pay the bills. Period. And that can put us in places we don't want, in jobs we don't want. Remember that with food, you can have cheesecake, as long as you eat it in moderation. Any food can be part of your dietary repertoire—you just need to know how to consume it. Anything you want to do as part of your work is also okay. This may mean that although you're currently a teacher, you want to sell your paintings. You may need to keep teaching to pay the bills, but your art is also your "work," and in fact may be your calling, so integrate it into your working life and allow it to become part of your occupational identity, even if you aren't getting paid for it yet. Paint at night and on weekends, and perhaps one day, you will find yourself painting full-time.

In the workplace, one of the issues that people often struggle with is the pursuit of a dream as a vocation. Too many people do not spend their days doing what they love for a living, or they do something for a long time and then decide at some point that it's not for them. Certainly, there are professions that are harder to enter or to get paid for—particularly creative pursuits. Many people will literally disavow the part of themselves that wants to do something else because it reminds them of something they left behind. I would argue that the two can coexist; you can be a plumber-poet, an accountant-accordionist, an administrator-actor, a salesman-snowboarder, a professor-pundit. Paying the rent doesn't mean you end the dream; the two are not mutually exclusive.

After I lost the weight and was able to walk away from a marriage, I figured what the hell, this spider-sense thing seems to be working out for me, so I will pursue a dream. But it would have to be a hybrid. As a single mom I would have to pay the bills, and thus, my academic job was still important to me. I just wanted something else. I had long wanted to pursue a career in the media and desperately wanted to write this book. Despite numerous people discouraging me, I was told about an agent who represented mental health people in the media. I sent him a snapshot and my résumé, and he agreed to meet with me.

I used a frequent-flier ticket and flew across the country and stayed on a friend's couch in New Jersey. I met with him and he thought I was sellable. Six months later I was working on a series on Bravo, started doing media commentary for a variety of news outlets, and a year later, a publisher bought my book. Three years ago I was told no, but I pushed past the fear. What was the worst that would happen? I would be laughed at? I would fail? What was more frightening to me was to never try. I now find the hybrid of my academic, writing, and television careers to be as satisfying a professional life as I could ever imagine, but it required listening to my spider senses to get to this place.

Think about ways you can find a balance between paying the bills and honoring what you want to do. If your dream is in an area totally foreign to your career, can you enjoy it as a hobby? Can you get up at dawn and spend time on it before you leave for work? Can you do it on weekends? Can you take a break from your job? Can you retrain in a new field? I'll bet the thought of even taking on your dream is overwhelming. Research has found that people who are oriented to the needs and wants of others (for example, going to law school because your father wanted you to) may struggle more with self-regulation and willpower than those who are honoring their own goals and hopes. This is consistent with the idea that silencing your spider senses in the service of your stakeholders actually makes it harder to accomplish things. It also speaks to an interesting connection between eating and working. If you are miserable at work and expending willpower just to get through the day, it's possible that you will have more difficulty saying no to food.

LISTENING TO YOUR SPIDER SENSES TO FIND THE RIGHT CAREER FOR YOU

Even more overwhelming may be the idea that you do not yet have a dream. I remember sitting at a children's park once with a woman who knew me peripherally and who praised me for the pursuit of my dream, but said, "I wouldn't know what to pursue; I don't even have a dream." I felt sad when I heard her say that, but I wondered how much she had silenced her inner voice lest she feel threatened by it. Give your dreams a chance to take flight. The beauty of the

If you are miserable at work and expending willpower just to get through the day, it's possible that you will have more difficulty saying no to food.

exercises in this book is that they are private. You can record anything; no one can judge what you write, and perhaps by engaging in the exercises, you may launch some of your dreams.

Many times we know we need to change how we eat and reduce our weight, but to do so means to change the status quo. And once we start changing the status quo in one place, it often results in shifts in other places. Change tends to generalize and, as noted in the chapter on relationships, once you start taking care of you and advocating for yourself through your health decisions, it is quite conceivable that you will also start advocating for yourself at work—or at least start exploring how to pursue work that is more of a calling than a chore.

This is also about being realistic. A young person cannot expect to walk into an entry-level job and get the corner office. Watch the career trajectories of those around you. Are people advancing, or are they stuck? Is it an industry where you need to continually switch employers? If people are advancing, why is it happening? Do you possess the characteristics of those in leadership within your organization? Perhaps it's the right industry but the wrong organization. The risk at work is to grow complacent, in fact, it is essential to always monitor, stay on top of trends, and be aware of what you want within your career and work world.

I have spoken to many people who had intense jobs in intense industries and prospered, but then one day it became too much, and they went on to fulfilling careers as volunteers, therapists, caterers, musicians, and boat makers. One of my favorite work-related spider-senses stories comes from an acquaintance who had a job in an industry he liked well enough, but who went on to become a professional poker player. He had no regrets about the transition despite protestations from stakeholders, the usual fears, and the golden rules. Interestingly, he made enough to live on for a while, then he had a cold streak, and his spider senses told him that he needed to create a hybrid occupation, so now he does some work in his original area of training to pull a steady paycheck while continuing the poker playing. (He himself acknowledged that trusting his gut was key at the poker table, and when he hit a rough patch, he knew he had to find a middle ground.)

STAKEHOLDERS, FEAR, AND LEAVING JOB SECURITY

Walking away from the workplace can be as challenging as walking away from relationships or any half-full plates in our lives. Stakeholders, fears, and golden rules play here as heavily as anywhere. Work is a strong part of our identity. A person may introduce him- or herself and say, "Hello, I'm John, I'm a teacher," or "I'm Julia, I'm a dentist." I know a friend who went speed-dating, having twenty, three-minute dates in one night. The question after "What's your name?" was "What do you do for a living?" Our careers become part of our identity and communicate something to the world about us. If we are doing work that is not congruent with who we are or what we want, it can be taxing to our sense of identity, and in some ways, a denial of our spider senses. If we are doing work we don't enjoy without some area of our life being fulfilled by pleasurable work or activities, it can be numbing—a bit like eating too much.

The idea of walking away from a job, especially what is considered to be a "good" job, can be met with significant consternation and worry by stakeholders. Stakeholders may directly be affected, especially if your departure from one job results in a change in financial resources or a change in status. I recently watched a dear friend leave an established, well-regarded position in his industry for something that would allow him to be more creative and potentially bring in more money but also carried far more risk. Out of the gate it may not have had the same prestige, but it would allow him to enact his vision. His stakeholders reacted strongly, panicky about the loss of revenue and security, and "Are you sure-d" him about the loss of prestige. He held his position and made the transition but definitely agonized over the choice. Honoring your spider senses can sometimes mean even more struggle, especially in the workplace, because there is often risk when you listen to spider senses.

His story speaks to the fact that heeding spider senses can be very scary, especially at work. Initially, things did not go smoothly; the voices of his stakeholders repeatedly caused him to question himself, and his fears grew because the new, risky project wasn't taking shape. He doubted himself. Yet, at a spider-sense level, he knew he did not want to go back to the old job, the place where his stakeholders had told him to stay. Finally, after holding on and pushing through the fear, the rewards of creating his own vision and honoring his voice quieted the stakeholders and magnified his spider senses. He now reports that his career is twice as rewarding as it ever was, and it has opened up new opportunities that are many times more financially rewarding than the "prestigious" job he held before.

Jobs are very much about security. Some jobs are steadier than others, and those that do not carry high risk are often quite comforting, even if they are unfulfilling, especially in a challenging economy. So it does become a challenging balance to avoid becoming numbed by a job while retaining your spider senses and vision. A difficult economy is its own form of stakeholder, because it requires us to make different kinds of decisions, and it is also a form of data. It may mean we won't quit one job to pursue another interest, or it may simply mean working harder to do the work we need and the work we want.

What are your fears of what will happen if you leave your job or change your career path? Homelessness? Poverty? Loss of status? Loss of stakeholders? Any of these things are possible, and I recognize that the challenging economic times in which we find ourselves means those of us who have jobs are often grateful. But that acceptance does not need to result in denying what you want—it may just mean working harder. Just like with eating, it is easy to work lazily and mindlessly. It takes effort to think about what you eat, just like it takes effort to think about your calling and what you want to do.

When we listen to ourselves, we can eat healthier. When we pay attention, we can make better decisions and practice better willpower. When we stop and take a moment to assess, we will not only gatekeep better in the workplace, but also figure out ways to either walk away or integrate what we want to do with what we already do.

GOLDEN RULES AND WORK

What are the golden rules you were taught about work? Work isn't fun? A good worker stays loyal to the same company? You are supposed to retire at age sixty-five? Were you raised by nine-to-five parents who worked in an office and still believe that any job you can do from home is not a "real job"? Were you told that creative pursuits are not real jobs? Jobs, like food and relationships, have early origins: Before we can walk or talk, parents are already projecting dreams onto us: Johnny is going to be a lawyer. Mary is going to be a doctor. One of the first things we are asked is, "What are you going to be when you grow up?" These early lessons set a script for us, as they do with food, which is hard to break. We are sometimes puppets when it comes to the types of careers our parents want for us.

When I work with parents of young adults, I tell them to allow their child to honor his or her spider senses and become who they truly want to be. They often bristle at the idea of their child—who just spent four years in college—taking a minimum-wage or unpaid job to pursue their dreams of being a musician or artist, or a poorly paid position as a production assistant with aspirations of being a director. My advice: Let them honor their spider senses; let them find their way. You don't have to underwrite the costs if you don't want to, but by letting them go through their own process, they can honor their voice. In some cases they may succeed brilliantly in their chosen field; others may shape it into something else; or, they may give it a shot, honor their spider senses, and then walk away. Do not dictate their path; it is no different than clipping their wings. Weigh in, give suggestions, but then let go. It is the most loving gesture of all. Try to refrain from asking, "Are you sure?"

GATEKEEPING AND YOUR CAREER

For the past thirteen years I've had the good fortune of working with college students as a university professor. In those years, I have worked with hundreds of students who are trying to figure out what to do with their lives, and I do my best to stave off gatekeeping disasters. Many students come in with their spider senses so scrambled that they might as well say, "My mother wants me to . . ." because they have no idea what they want for themselves.

Once the appointment is over they usually leave far more confused than they were when they entered, but a new conversation has begun nonetheless. Some leave galvanized with the drive and perhaps greater certainty that they want to become a psychologist; others leave and start a new process of self-exploration. What concerns me is that they tend to put their heads down and attempt to live to a formula rather than really take a moment and ask themselves what they want their lives to look like. I even tell them that it's okay to want money; they just need to know that about themselves so they can make the best possible choices. Instead of judging ourselves, we need to let ourselves run free. When I meet with undergraduates, I ask them to figure out what all the other people in their world want for them and then separate it from what *they* want. I have taken what I typically do with my undergraduates and have turned it into an exercise whereby you can do some of the same exploration.

EXERCISE: ASSESSING THE JOB YOU WANT VERSUS THE JOB YOU HAVE

Breaking it down:

- What is your current profession? (*Unemployed* is a perfectly fine answer here.)

- What are you trained to do?

- Can you make enough to live on your current salary?

- How do you want to spend your days?

- Are you doing what you want to be doing?

Much like with a plate of food, you need to listen to your spider senses to determine if you are "full" at your job. Think about when you're not hungry and you keep eating anyway. The food usually doesn't taste very good, yet you keep on eating. It's a bit like that at work; the work isn't very rewarding, yet you keep on working. Always keeping in mind that it may not be economically expedient to leave a job, it is important to figure out how to build your calling into your day.

Are you full? Would you rather be doing something else, maybe something you've always dreamt of? If yes, then you have an entirely longer set of questions to answer for yourself. First you have to slow down and listen to your spider senses, because you need to really address what you want to do with your life, professionally, and figure out its feasibility economically.

Make a plan: Can you figure out how to spend your time doing what you want to do while still being able to pay the bills? Can you do it part-time if not full-time?

Mindfully collect data: Talk to mentors, career advisors, friends, and people in similar lines of work. The mindful part comes from the fact that many may discourage you (it happened to me left and right during my journey—I would listen to them and integrate their feedback, but never let them pull me off my path). The discouraging advice of others does not have to push you off your path; instead, it can warn you of pitfalls and galvanize you to fight harder. There's nothing like a call to arms before taking on a new challenge.

The Promise of One: If you can pull this off—and you know you can—then enact the Promise of One. Practice by listening to yourself and each day doing one thing to get closer to that goal. It may be contacting someone in the field, filling out a school application, or checking your bank balance.

THE WHY

We spend a significant part of our adult lives at our jobs, and a life spent in a miserable job can all but destroy our spider senses. Even in a tough economy when any job seems like a good job, there are ways to heed your spider senses to make your current job into something you like, push through the fear, take risks, and consider doing something new.

What are some signs that you are "full" from your job and that you may need to either walk away or find something new to complement your work life? Answer the following questions:

- Has the quality of your work diminished? Are you missing deadlines? Is the quality of the product you deliver suffering? Are others noticing this?

- Do you dread going to work, and find yourself wishing you didn't have to go?

- Do you spend time thinking about other jobs, careers, or going back to school?

- Do you use work time inefficiently, and regularly resent having to complete the responsibilities of your job?

- Are you bored, and do work activities that used to give you pleasure (or at least satisfaction) no longer do so?

- Are you missing days, calling in sick, using personal days, or just plain playing hooky?

- Do you feel unhappy more days than you feel happy at work (really weigh this one—is it all the time, or some of the time)?

It feels analogous to having trouble with a relationship, or life in general. When you no longer enjoy your work   you're phoning it in, you want to be somewhere else, and you derive little pleasure from it—then your job becomes a chore. It becomes necessary to either walk away or reshape the context of your work life.

THE NOW

I want you to complete two exercises now.

Career Check-Up

The first is a sort of "job diagnosis," so grab your journal and record the following:

- What do you want your professional life to look like?

- What is your current job?

- Rate your job satisfaction on a 1-to-10 scale (1 is completely dissatisfied, 10 completely satisfied). What would you need to make your job a 10?

- List five things you would change about your job (more if you want).

- List five things you love about your job (more if you want).

- What do your stakeholders feel about your job?

- What are your fears if you leave?

- How did you come to this job?

- What do your spider senses tell you?

- What do you want to be when you grow up?

Labors of Love

For the second exercise, list the ten jobs or tasks you would never want. Next list ten jobs or tasks you dream of doing (it can be more if you want, less if you want as well). Your list could read: professional skydiver, guitarist, writer, mechanic, life coach. Think big and don't edit yourself as you go. Just write the list as it pops into your head.

List five to ten structural things you need or want from a job (minimum salary, flexibility, office, travel, and so on).

Okay, now let's analyze your answers a bit. By that I mean you might have written down basketball player, but at the age of fifty, it's a little late in the game to join the NBA. However, you could coach a youth league, join a regular pickup game, train as a referee, or write a basketball blog.

Say you want to become a writer; let's look at some steps you can take to achieve this dream. If you want to be a writer but you're a full-time personal assistant, can you take a class after work once a week to see what kind of writing you'd like to do? Can your company pay for the classes? You can't quit your day job and just sit at a computer and write— not just yet. But you can enact the Promise of One, and do one thing a day (or a week) to push yourself toward that goal. Can you find time to do what you love (even early in the morning or late at night)?

———◦‣———

Now, the assessment might take some time, and I want to be clear about something: I am not advocating that you quit your job and just go for it. You need a financial plan, a road map. So let's do this now. When you're trying to lose weight, looking down the pike at eighty pounds can overwhelm you, make you think you'll never get there, and ruin your ability to do it. But if you plot out ten-pound goals, it is easier. It's the same with finding a new job or career—it may feel impossible at first, but when you break it down into smaller, more-manageable steps, it becomes more feasible.

Let's assume you know you want to become a life coach. You're going to school part-time, you are working toward marketing yourself, and you know how you'll approach getting clients. Let's map out the money. How much start-up money do you need? This may depend on whether you are caring for a family or have to pay rent or a mortgage. At a minimum, figure out what it costs you to live for six to twelve months, and consider whether it's possible to save that ahead of time.

What can you sacrifice from your household budget to get there? Can you take a part-time job once school is finished, in addition to your day job, to build the cushion? Will you need a part-time job to keep afloat while starting your new venture?

Map it out. Write it down. You might not be able to execute your plan for two years, but just like my patient (the one I urged to plan a vacation she thought she could never afford), once you see it all on paper, you might be able to get there. She did with her trip. Use the Promise of One to keep your vision alive.

CHECK-IN: YOUR JOB

How do you identify yourself? Say it, and it will be so. After you've signed up to coach a Little League team, when asked "What do you do?" say, "I coach Little League part-time." The first time you write something—even if it's just for the local paper—when asked "What do you do?" you can try out your new identity and say, "I'm a writer." Don't say, "I'm a secretary, but I'm really struggling to become a writer. I just wrote a story for the local paper, so I hope I can write full-time very soon." No; the second you start to execute your plan, you've achieved a big part of your goal. Rewrite your story, and redefine who you are.

CHAPTER 15

Retail Therapy

Like so many Americans, she was trying to construct a life that made sense from things she found in gift shops.

—Kurt Vonnegut

I have worked with patients who overspend and overshop, and I've worked with clients on television who had a variety of shopping problems. As Dr. Ramani on the Oxygen series, *My Shopping Addiction,* I've had the opportunity to force people to face down their shopping issues through a variety of exercises. One theme emerged with every shopper on the show: Shopping was filling another need or distracting them from a larger problem—loneliness, anger, family discord, or unrealized dreams.

Many times we are trapped in a job because we are bingeing on something other than food—overshopping or overspending. Shopping has many of the same characteristics as eating. It is rewarding, numbing, distracting, and time-consuming. People who are shoppers typically use shopping as a tool for maintaining a certain profile in the world, or to distract themselves from a larger problem. Just like food, filling up on "stuff" can numb our spider senses.

Overspending can imprison us, too. People who shop are often in debt, have high mortgages, buy homes and rent storage units to hold their stuff, and are forced to work ever and ever harder to pay for these purchases. If you look at older homes, look at how much smaller their closets are compared to new construction. We are building houses and garages to house objects rather than people.

Kathleen Vohs and Ronald Faber, professors of marketing and mass communication at the University of Minnesota, have consistently pointed out in their work that willpower depletion affects shoppers. The more self-control shoppers have to exert in other areas of their lives, the more likely they are to splurge while shopping; just like with eating (and everything else), willpower can get depleted and lead to overspending. So if you're in a rotten job that depletes you, then you are more likely to spend money on more items and keep yourself stuck in a financial rut. Eventually, though, something will have to give.

Shopping has many of the same characteristics as eating. It is rewarding, numbing, distracting, and time-consuming.

GATEKEEPING CAN HELP YOU RESIST SPENDING TEMPTATIONS

So much of shopping is gatekeeping. Gatekeeping—not buying in the first place, or buying wisely and honoring your spider senses when it comes to finances and what shopping really brings you—can help you with this. The best way to avoid acquiring unnecessary stuff is to not go into the store in the first place. I understand that the world in which we live has not made this easy. Destination malls are a fortress of temptation. Here are some tips:

- Don't get in the car.
- Find other things to do that you enjoy to substitute for shopping.
- Don't carry credit cards with you if you do find yourself at a store.

We used to just have catalog shopping and QVC to resist. Now, with online shopping, it's possible to cave in to 2 a.m. shopping temptations. Here are a couple of tips to help you when you find the urge to splurge in your pajamas:

- Spending all that money may be keeping you from other loftier dreams. Put a Post-it on the computer(s) from which you shop to remind yourself what you are really sacrificing by purchasing that new jacket.

- Stick with debit cards instead of credit cards, so you are limited in your spending. Link that debit card to an account that is solely designated for discretionary spending, so you can't overspend.

FIGHT THE BUNKER MENTALITY

Another issue is what I call "bunker mentality," and it gets reinforced by advertisers, marketers, and Hollywood, in the form of shows where contestants attempt to "out-coupon" each other, or more cleverly purchase bargains. These people have the unique ability (and enough free time) to purchase hundreds or thousands of dollars' worth of merchandise and, by using coupons, spend nothing. At the end of it they still have lots of stuff—more stuff than a normal family can use.

Stocking up is one of the biggest rationales I hear for overspending and shopping. There are few things we cannot live without, and most of those things can be acquired at minimal cost, or improvised (soap, toilet paper, and clean water). We are not living in frontier America. If you need basic groceries (e.g. milk, butter, bread), you can probably get them quickly. (If you happen to live in a remote area and this isn't true for you, my apologies.) But when we see a "bargain," we feel compelled to spend time and resources to acquire it, even if we don't need it. Thus, you are wasting the present moment (and resources) on toilet paper or a giant case of juice you may not use for three months or ever.

The danger of stock-up shopping for eating habits is obvious, and can drown out your spider senses. You may want to take advantage of the cut-rate food and eat even when you're not hungry, just to get the "full bargain," but this is a misplaced frugality. When you purchase a gallon of mayonnaise or four pounds of pretzels, you feel compelled to consume them. Big-box stores that force you to buy larger quantities are in fact cheaper per ounce, because you are buying in bulk. But here's the rub: Will you consume every ounce? Maybe the better question is, *Should* you consume every ounce? Unless you have a family of twenty or are feeding a bunch of firefighters, I find it hard to rationalize big-box shopping. You tend to buy things you don't need because there's a good deal, or you buy more than you should and then consume it all. Sound familiar? Sounds a bit like those dirty plates that are so hard to walk away from.

Everybody loves a bargain, but these bargains are an illusion. If the gallon of mayonnaise costs $6 and a pint of mayonnaise costs $2, yes, ounce for ounce that gallon costs less. But that $4 savings carries lots of opportunity costs, including space and additional food consumption (because you feel compelled to eat it before it goes bad). And also, if you are buying in larger quantities, you may end up with less dietary variety, and that can lead to boredom at the dinner table and mindless overeating. Finally, big-box stores, because they are selling warehoused food, sell food that is processed to the hilt. Is that really what you want to take in day after day?

Remember what I said about treating your body like it deserves to be treated? I don't think eating endless frozen (processed) entrees is consistent with that philosophy. Savings do not just come down to dollars and cents; you need to take a longer view. Some people argue with me and say that big-box stores are the place to get certain items like wine and detergent. The problem is that given the depleted willpower most of us have, and our inability to walk away from the temptations that the big-box store offers, we walk in for trash bags and walk out with a new television and eight pounds of cookies.

When you think about shopping and eating, they're really quite similar. It's hard to walk away from a sale (like a half-full plate), even if you don't have the money or you don't need the items you are buying. We convince ourselves that we can shove in one more, and while it may not make us literally overweight, all that stuff is pouring over the edges of our drawers and closets, like our waistlines in our jeans. Just like you would relish a few really tasty bits on a plate if you ate mindfully and slowly, you may appreciate objects more if you are not drowning in them.

My executive producer on the shopping show said his grandmother often opined, "You can go broke saving money." She is dead-on. Once again we return to attention, monitoring, and mindfulness. One exercise that I often use with people who struggle with shopping is need and want. What do you need and what do you want? Do you need another new purse if you already have fifty? Do you need a new computer—or do you want one? If you are so flush that you can buy whatever you want, well, more power to you, but you need to keep in mind that shopping also requires time, and that is a resource more precious than money. All of that shopping can pull you away from the moment.

Invariably, people who struggle with shopping often manifest one other "habit"—smoking, overeating, drinking, or hoarding. The shopping tends to occur in a context of other blinding and numbing behaviors. Because the shopping is used to fill another "hole," it's not surprising that other things are used in the same way. Often it's a problem with walking away.

Here are some big-box rules to live by:

- Avoid them if you can. The savings aren't that astonishing when you take into account what you waste, or the boredom of repeatedly eating the same thing. When you walk in to get that one well-priced item, you will invariably spend more than you intend (the stores are designed for that), and walk out with stuff that is likely not good for your wallet or your waistline.

- If you have to go in, take a list and stick to it. Like eating mindfully, shop mindfully. Talk yourself through it if you must, and make that list on the basis of taking stock of your home. The apocalypse is not coming; you don't really need 100 rolls of toilet paper. And if it does come, my guess is that toilet paper will not be your primary concern.

- Share. If you can do this with others and separate the purchases, it can be cost-effective, but this does take some organization and coordination.

FEAR AND SPENDING

Have you ever been in a store and felt anxious that you would never find the item again, especially at that price? What would happen if you couldn't find it again? This is where our fears play a role: Fear can make us feel like we can't live without an item, or that we would regret it forever if we didn't get it. You may obsess about it for an hour, and those feelings are uncomfortable. If you can push through the anxiety and tolerate the discomfort, that is the first step to mastery and not giving in to the fears and, subsequently, the spending.

SPIDER SENSES AND SPENDING

Do you want it or need it? Spider senses play a role here, too. If shopping or purchasing that item makes you uncomfortable, because it will take an economic toll that you cannot afford, you will feel it in your gut. Buyer's remorse is merely your spider senses saying "Probably not." There are times when your spider senses may tell you that a certain purchase represents a rare opportunity, but take a step back and take stock of whether you are getting a deal or trying to fill some other need. A new dress feels good for a night, but if you are struggling with other holes in your life, that dress will only be a temporary fix, and may have bigger ramifications in terms of finances.

Spending can also spiral into much larger purchases. Some of us dig ourselves into holes with mortgages, car loans, and the rest of it. Whether it is window dressing or distraction, it can set you up for a life where you are working to keep up the facade rather than living. I have seen so many people make exquisite sacrifices to purchase a home—move far away from the people they love, get second jobs they do not like or want, work longer hours—and then they are away from the very family and friends they hoped to invite over to their new home. Somehow the illusion of the house and the idea that it would somehow complete them kept them going. When making any purchase—big-ticket or not—stop and listen to those spider senses.

STAKEHOLDERS AND SPENDING

Stakeholders definitely play a role in our spending habits. Stakeholders can tell us that we need that dress, look great in that car, or should settle down and buy a house. They set the bar, too, perhaps sneering at our label-less clothes. Stakeholders and society feed us with ideals about the right car, right address, and all the right stuff, and they set up an aspirational vision of homes that look like Pottery Barn catalogs. At such times our spider senses are rendered numb as we try to figure out what we want. When it comes to spending, the media has us by the throat, and it takes tremendous fortitude to resist. The media has given us a script that says designer clothes, fancy cars, the right gadget, and the right sofa are the fast track to happiness. It's hard to listen to yourself in the midst of that din.

In my work with people who can't stop the shopping, especially the high-end shopping, it is often about maintaining an image that is not consistent with reality. I have had women tell me that even if they are broke, that if they carry a $3,000 purse then people will assume they are somehow important or successful. When people are so driven by what the stakeholders think, it is easy to lose sight of our inner voice and start living and spending for others, rather than inherently valuing ourselves.

Data can help you make better decisions that align with your spider senses and ignore the voices of the stakeholders. What kinds of data are useful when shopping? What do you really need? Make lists based on an inventory of your home and your budgetary limits, and use this data to make responsible spending decisions. Then take a step back and let your spider senses do their thing.

BAD MONEY AFTER GOOD

We do it at the dinner table, we do it in our relationships, and we even do it at the casino; why wouldn't we do it at the store? We often throw bad money after good. What does that mean? Just like we find it hard to leave leftovers at the restaurant or food on our plates, it doesn't feel good to leave the store empty-handed. Many shoppers I have worked with have talked about how walking out of a store without a bag feels empty, sad, and pointless, so they sometimes spend to avoid that feeling. If we go in and can't find the thing we want, it can be hard to walk away empty-handed because we've already invested the time, the parking, the effort (sounds a bit like marriage doesn't it?). Stay on top of this common error. Remember, as I said earlier, research has shown that we make more impulse buys the longer we are at it, and the more overwhelmed we are by choices. Sometimes shopping is just a day out of the house, people-watching and researching our options. But spending money just for the sake of spending it, because you invested the time, is like cleaning your plate because you paid for it.

THE WHY

Spending is like eating; it makes us feel better. But let's be clear—just like when you overeat, there are consequences: You gain weight. If you overspend, you drop into a terrible cycle of debt and that might not only mean you have two big problems, but also you could suddenly have more. Shopping also takes time—time away from other people, time that could be spent nourishing yourself in a better way. You might find debt stressful and overeat to manage that stress. Don't create more problems for yourself by spending. It's like chocolate cake—it only feels good for a moment. How many pairs of shoes are enough?

THE NOW

Take stock of what you do have at home. Most of us never do that, and it's a powerful exercise. Socks, underwear, soap, butter—you name it. You will be surprised at how much stuff you have, and you may make some interesting discoveries.

Purge. If you haven't worn it in a year, lose it. Give it to charity or make a buck and consign it. If you didn't wear it much, don't get another.

Follow these shopping tips:

- Learn to differentiate between want and need. We are socialized by a covetous media to want, but there is little that we need. When you reach for something in the store, or even spend time shopping, reflect on that.

- Put it down, walk away, and come back in a day. Some decisions need a moment to percolate. The car will still be there tomorrow; so, too, will the sofa or whatever it is you wanted to buy. I am guessing that 75 percent of the time, you won't go back and purchase the item.

- Make a list and stick to it.

- Distract yourself. If you go shopping, you are going to spend money and time. If you go into a restaurant, you are going to eat. So don't even enter the store (or the restaurant) in the first place. Do something else—see a friend, take a walk, go to a movie.

- Curb the carbs and the cards. If you do go shopping, don't carry your credit cards with you, and allot yourself a certain amount of cash. This is a bit like using a smaller plate. You can only pile so much food up on a small plate, and you can only spend so much money if you have a fixed amount.

- Don't shop hungry. We know that depleted willpower leads to a harder time self-controlling while shopping, so make sure you are well fed when you enter a store; otherwise you may start binge-spending.

PROMISE OF ONE

You can take back your shopping habits one day at a time. Some suggestions include making a budget, cleaning out a closet and giving away a bag of clothes, and cutting up and canceling a credit card. One thing a day can help clear the clutter and allow you to unbury yourself from the stuff and the spending.

CHECK-IN: SHOPPING

Is there a dream that you have postponed because it is too expensive? Perhaps a trip or a tool to help you with a hobby, like a new camera? Force yourself to save for it, and that means shopping less. Take a moment and determine what you want—then get it. How much do you need to set aside each week? Implement the Promise of One. It can help if you see that your sacrifice is advancing you toward your larger goal.

PART FOUR:

Taking Risks and Learning to Fly

CHAPTER 16

The Body Count

The most painful thing in life is losing yourself in the process of valuing someone too much and forgetting that you are special too.

—Buddhist text

This is it. This is where the rubber meets the road. This is why you don't face the fears, walk away from the plate, or the relationship, or the job: the body count.

If you do what you know is right for you, if you listen to yourself, then you worry that people will leave you.

And guess what? They will.

I am not going to sugarcoat that.

It's difficult, but I'd like you to listen to the darker side of your spider senses, pushing past those fears and taking on your stakeholders. Until now spider senses have been all good—taking you to a life you want. However, these losses are real, and there are ways to cope with and perhaps even avoid them—or at least, to soften them. I have often been told by patients, friends, and family that it's okay to pursue your happiness as long as nobody gets hurt. That's a cop-out. If you pursue your authentic self, trust your spider senses, and do what feels right for you, you *will* disappoint others, and many will feel threatened and possibly hurt. If you are surrounded by people who want the best for you, even if it is disruptive for them, count yourself among the lucky, because most of us are not.

Healthy weight loss teaches us to move past this fear of disappointment and awaken our spider senses. We are then more likely to become better gatekeepers, which can make things less messy but also lead us to take greater risks. That can be unsettling for those around us.

George Bernard Shaw summed up the body count beautifully when he stated, "If you begin by sacrificing yourself to those you love, you will end by hating those to whom you have sacrificed yourself." Read on to learn how to face the body count, manage it, and, ultimately, perhaps save some relationships by honoring yourself first.

A CAUTIONARY TALE

This is a story of a wealthy couple from the East Coast. He was a successful entrepreneur, and she was a stay-at home mother. She was young when they married, yet her family heartily supported the union. The groom was wealthy and from a socially prominent family; the bride's entire family would experience a social boost and lots of goodies from this marriage. Their cultural background was such that this marriage would suit both families well, and if she hadn't followed through with it, her family would have been disappointed—and she knew it. She didn't finish her college degree because her new husband said, "Why would you need it? I will take care of you forever." The young woman and her husband purchased a large estate and threw lavish parties. Her parents became the toast of the town and were thrilled to be along for the ride. The young couple quickly went on to have children, and for a while, the wealth, the activity, and the children distracted everyone from what was unfolding.

She was not happy. She never really had been, and reported that she'd had misgivings from the very beginning. She confessed to getting caught up in the fairy-tale wedding and the lifestyle; it was wonderful to have everyone—parents, grandparents, community—fawning over her. Other young women wanted to be her. For a while, the designer clothes, the vacations, the cars, and the full social calendar distracted from the issue at hand. But her husband was a bit of a tyrant, controlling and demanding, and as she started to make friends outside of her cultural social circle, she found that she was not comfortable with how her husband treated her. All the purses and shoes in the world wouldn't change that.

When she challenged him, he reacted coldly, angrily, and sometimes dangerously. There was tension at home, and her children were anxious and fearful. When she shared her misgivings with her family, community members, and some friends, they told her she was acting like a "spoiled child"; that she was "irresponsible and selfish" for wanting to leave a marriage that had given her so much material comfort. So she stuck it out and over time it got sloppy—infidelities and violence ensued. Ultimately, despite the protests of everyone, she decided to listen to her spider senses and leave.

What was the body count? Pretty substantial. Her parents disowned her, calling her every name in the book. Most of her extended family disavowed her. Her in-laws threatened legal action for all kinds of unfounded reasons. Her entire community cut her out of their events. Her children experienced substantial distress. Friends they had shared during the marriage bid her farewell. Her ex-husband put her through a legal hell, with lawyers' fees in the millions. He threatened her, and she endured significant health problems as a result. It was what she had been afraid of, and the reason why she'd put it off.

As a rule we avoid things that we fear. Ironically, she put off the inevitable and she suffered additional needless years in her marriage, living in fear of these reactions. When she finally pulled the trigger and left, she had to tolerate the body count anyhow. Are you wondering what happened to her? Let's take a look at what the body count was, and then we'll see how it turned out.

THE FOOD BODY COUNT

Does this really relate to food? Yes. Think about your dinner-table stakeholders, the people who want you to order a certain way, eat a certain way, and actually eat a certain amount. You can either (a) keep them in your life, and give in to their demands; (b) keep them in your life and communicate your discomfort with how you feel about their comments (which could lead to fights, but also some good discourse); or (c) do what you feel to be right and let the chips fall where they may (that means you tolerate the discomfort of others).

I have one patient who is unwilling to incur the body count of losing her in-laws, major contributors to her challenges with food. The strategy she has crafted is to eat healthily and listen to her spider senses at all times when she is not with them, and when she is with them, she succumbs to their demands. It is not a perfect solution because their issues bleed into her regular days at the table, but at least she is aware of their contribution.

LOSING SOME STAKEHOLDERS, GAINING BETTER ONES

The hardest step is the first one—taking the risk and acknowledging the potential losses. We are so afraid of change, of rejection, of upsetting the apple cart, of the body count, that we avoid making a step, making a choice, or walking away. One way to manage this is to do what I call "stealth" change. The idea of making a big change and facing down everyone may seem too big, so starting quietly and slowly may be a way to take on the body count.

Some people never came back into my life after my journey and life changes—a sobering tale of how tenuous those relationships were to begin with. However, when you clear out, you make room for the new. Some folks came back, and we do a cautious dance of rebuilding trust. Most joyous were the new people who came into my life. With the courage, authenticity, and strength came better gatekeeping for new relationships and unconditional stakeholders. My life is now populated by such people, and no matter what I tell them—no matter how outlandish—they smile and love me and let me make my mistakes and celebrate my failures. And they don't care when I refuse a second helping.

What about body counts that get reduced—people who leave us and then come back? You are not returning to the original relationship. They showed you what they were made of, and in that moment in time, they didn't trust you or stand by you. Once they got more data or moved past it, they came back. Can you forgive them? That's a personal decision. Can you forget? Not a good idea.

Consider Desmond Tutu's thoughts on forgiveness: "Forgiving is not forgetting; it's actually remembering—remembering and not using your right to hit back. It's a second chance for a new beginning. And the remembering part is particularly important. Especially if you don't want to repeat what happened." Don't forgive blindly, and use the data to move forward into newly strengthened relationships and new relationships.

After the body count gets reduced and some people return, you'll find that you are entering newly rendered relationships. You may be more cautious in these new spaces because what was done to you once may very likely be done to you again. You can now consume these people in a more-informed way. Do they laugh every time you tell them a dream? Stop telling them your dreams.

PREPARE FOR BACKLASH

Don't marry just for the wedding, or to cave to stakeholders,
but expect criticism and chiding.

Don't stay in a job just to avoid a difficult situation with your parents,
but expect them to express their disappointment.

Don't stay married for the children, the friends, or the house,
but expect that people may distance themselves from you, and that your children will be very upset.

Don't eat for the waiter,
but expect that he or she may look at you in a way that will make you feel guilty.

Don't go to college because "That's what people do after high school" (I realize this is a somewhat controversial statement, considering I am a college professor, but I can say confidently, college is not for everyone. We're conditioned to think we must send our kids to college, and that to achieve success we ourselves must attend and graduate. But we're all wired just a little bit differently, and there is no shame in career paths that don't require a traditional college education; in fact, I know that many plumbers make more money than professors),
but expect that people will warn you that you "may not look good on paper" if you skip doing this.

CHOOSE YOUR DREAM CATCHERS CAREFULLY

It's amazing to me how cavalier we are with our dreams, particularly new dreams, ideas, or ventures. We just share them with other people, wagging our tails and tongues like puppies as we wait for the other person to get as excited as we are. The fact is that most people are not good dream catchers. Their own issues get in the way of being authentic and enthusiastic cheerleaders for their friends and family, which can be lethal to us, our dreams, and our vision. Dreams are like children. For those of you who are parents or pet owners, this will ring true. We are typically careful to vet the qualifications and/or reputation of any person with whom we will leave our children or animals. We take great pains to choose people known to us and our kids, or people with certain credentials. You may enjoy spending endless weekend hours with your drinking buddies, but you may not entrust your loved ones to them because it may not be in the kids' or pets' best interest.

The same should apply to your dreams. Entrusting your dreams or aspirations to the wrong person could be a critical mistake, lest they mistreat or neglect them. We are not nearly as careful with our dreams as we should be.

Here's the takeaway that you must remember: Your success means different things to different people, and while others may not be consciously holding you back or hurting that embryonic idea of yours, some people just don't like change, some are resentful, and some are angry about the dreams they gave up.

Entrusting your dreams or aspirations to the wrong person could be a critical mistake, lest they mistreat or neglect them. We are not nearly as careful with our dreams as we should be.

The reasons are myriad but the outcome is the same. When that unformed dream is laughed at, questioned, or belittled, it may not recover. Worse, you may scrap the whole thing altogether.

THE BODY COUNT AND FEAR

In life, if you heed your spider senses, you are going to hurt people, but avoiding doing that at the expense of yourself, well, that's an easy out. If you pursue your happiness, your voice, and what you want, people are going to get hurt. If you live your life in the service of not hurting others, you will incur losses yourself. At some level, everyone around you is trying to keep their world comfortable, so if your decision inserts a change into their lives, they may fight it. Now, not everyone is like this, and when you find people who are supportive, hold on tight, because they are relatively rare. These people will let you do what you need even if it means change or challenge for them. More troublesome are the people who make it clear what they expect from you and the choices they want you to make. You may very well be holding back on some big-ticket decisions because of their discomfort. Guess what? They will not congratulate or celebrate you for choosing as they wish, but the first time you do something they don't want, they will castigate you for going against them.

At the end of your life, do you want to look back and say you shelved your dreams and ignored your voice and lived as others wanted you to? Or do you want to look back on your own life, mistakes and all, and know it was yours? Both choices carry implications. Can you do this without hurting people? You can certainly do things to minimize it. Be honest and open about who you are and what you want, early and often.

COMMUNICATE TO MANAGE THE BODY COUNT

Here is where communication may be your only tool to help manage body counts before and after they happen. Here are some tips:

Keep the lines of communication open—don't tamp down discomforts and be inauthentic in the name of keeping peace.

Be open and honest in how you talk to others. Honesty doesn't mean cruelty. But sometimes delaying honesty can result in even greater cruelty.

Gatekeep and be careful at the beginning, and you will be less likely to bring into your life people who will become part of a body count. The fact is, avoiding a body count and focusing on not hurting others is the ultimate cop-out, because it allows you to not take responsibility for your own choices, or lack thereof. You may look like a martyr to the world for sacrificing your life in the name of keeping others happy, but then you never need to take the chances and bold risks that characterize living authentically, honestly, and in line with your spider senses. There are those people who are there from the beginning—family and folks you don't choose. Most people don't wake up in the morning wanting to hurt people. We want to support our networks and have them support us. So when what we want to do is at odds with what they want—whether it is not taking a second helping of what they cooked for us, or making a career change that they do not support—it's then that we often make our worst choices in the name of trying to avoid a body count.

Prepare your stakeholders for what you are going to do, then do it. Make the communication about you (I feel, I want), and don't hurl insults.

I worked with a client who was spending all of her time and money shopping, and she would often end up with five of the same item because she had so much stuff and had lost track of it all. Instead of eating, she shopped, but it had the same effect—it wasted time and money. She had good rationalizations for it: She was a bargain shopper, so she would reflect on her great bargains, her special style, and the satisfaction she received. She wasn't going into debt, so what did it matter?

However, when we dug below the surface, it turned out that there were some deeper issues. She had left school and was in an evening job that had little future. Her family had discouraged her from pursuing her dreams of a career in fashion or music, saying, "Everyone wants to do that; you have no chance of succeeding." She did not feel that she could speak out against her family, who had already experienced so many struggles, but she also couldn't see herself taking on the career they wanted for her. So she was stuck, and she shopped to distract herself from what she was really giving up in the name of avoiding a body count.

Once we connected the dots between the blind shopping and the blind living, she got it. Unfortunately, she was still too scared to make changes, and could not imagine facing down her family and telling them her truth. So we broke it down further and used the Promise of One. She did her one call, one e-mail, one thing a day. She wound up getting an internship, finding an affordable course of study for what she wants to do, and slowly giving up the shopping habit. If she had just tried to stop the shopping without understanding *why* she was shopping, it would have been too much; if she had tried to talk to her family, they would have dissuaded her. Taking it on little by little makes it manageable.

Keep the lines of communication open—don't tamp down discomforts and be inauthentic in the name of keeping peace. Be open and honest in how you talk to others.

Even after all this communicating and doing things organically and quietly, might there still be a body count? Yes. But armed with the momentum of the changes you are making, one day at a time, you are already in the midst of it and have the strength to face down your fears and just keep doing it.

BEING SELFISH

You are selfish. How dare you? These are not easy things to hear. Many people who get a divorce are termed selfish. People who work long and hard on a dream are often considered selfish. People who may choose to take time for themselves are often labeled selfish. Let's think about the word *selfish,* which is defined in *Merriam-Webster's Collegiate Dictionary* as "seeking or concentrating on one's own advantage, pleasure, or well-being without regard for others." Ouch! We need a word for just the first part: "seeking or concentrating on one's . . . pleasure or well-being." Most of us who do this struggle and work hard to find a balance. But stakeholders use the world *selfish* like a double-barreled shotgun to keep us from making any changes and rocking the boat.

————◄○►————

What about our lady of the bad marriage and the big house? Her parents finally witnessed one of her husband's verbally violent attacks, and once they had directly observed him, they came around. Her siblings and many cousins, aunts, and uncles observed his actions, and they came around. Her children, no longer living in a situation characterized by distress and hostility, came around. The friends they shared during the marriage chose to stick by him and never came around. Her community was split, and half of them never returned. The parents of her children's friends didn't want to be involved in a "scandal," and so most never came back, or else they put on a face of doing so and continued whispering behind her back.

Her body count was high. But in speaking with her recently, she shared that she was at peace for the first time in her life. She realized that the fear of losing everyone was terrifying and had taken her to some dark places, but once it happened, it wasn't so bad. Because in its place came new people—different kinds of stakeholders who stood by her no matter what, a man who loves her unconditionally, and children who are finally relaxed and happy. She doesn't miss the folks who left her; in fact, she moved away to a different area and no longer has to endure their stares in public places.

Some bodies come back to life and some do not. You may be wondering if this is a happy ending. I think it is an *authentic* ending, and that is the best ending of all. Heeding your spider senses becomes truth serum, and, sadly, a test of the relationships around you. If honoring you results in the loss of a relationship, it is a litmus test that such a relationship was in fact conditional (a relationship in which the other person says, "Do what I want, and everything will be fine"). It's a great way to weed out the people who are only there for themselves.

THE WHY

Body counts will happen when you listen to your spider senses, but communication is one of our best and most respectful tools to help prepare those around us for the changes we need to make, to exert what we want, and also to ensure that new stakeholders are clear on who we are and what we want.

Forgiveness is not forgetting. After the body count, when people come back to you, it's okay to welcome them back; just be wise, and be aware of how to best consume them. The corollary here is that while neither of you may be able to forget the past, you also should not live in it, and if the newly rendered relationship consists of having old hurts being pushed back and forth, reassess.

You are only as good as your last meal. Human beings are not bank accounts. We like to think that if we do ten good things and just one bad thing, the ten good things will cancel out the one bad. It doesn't work that way, because people remember the last thing you did. So think hard about holding off on making an essential change because you don't want to anger them. They will be angry, but what's the worst thing that will happen? There is also a corollary to this. People have short memories, and absence makes the heart grow fonder. More often than you think, people forgive. Sadly, many people hold off on making big decisions for years because they don't want to anger someone. Waiting won't stop that, and if anything, it will give you more years to heal in the wake of the other person's anger and move forward into a bright new future.

Sticks and stones. Many people are afraid of being called names and being rejected. Again—what is the worst thing that could happen? The insults are just words, and if you are living a life that is yours, such words have little power.

Anxiety leads us to avoid. In our fear of having a showdown with a stakeholder or of being laughed at or discouraged, we feel anxious, and subsequently either postpone the conversation or the change we need to make. Anxiety is a spider-sense scrambler—it's like taking a cell phone through a tunnel. You want that signal back? Push through the tunnel and listen to yourself and your spider senses again.

THE NOW

This is a communication exercise that starts with you. Think about the people in your life with whom you are not communicating as clearly as you could, or where this lack of clarity may be setting you up for some big problems. List them out and make clear for yourself what you want to say to them. For example, you may want to talk to your spouse or partner about a career change you hope to make, or talk with a supervisor about taking on some extra shifts at work.

First, jot down your fears about what would happen if you approached them.

Second, think of what you want to say to them, in a best-case world, and then practice it with a friend. Find someone you trust (preferably an unconditional stakeholder or therapist) and just say it out loud.

Why will this help you? Just getting those words out may make you ready to say them aloud when you have the opportunity to converse with that person. Remember, you may not be able to avoid the body count, but you may be able to soften it.

Are you holding back on your dreams? Assess the body count. Many times people refrain from aspirations or opportunities—anything ranging from weight loss to job change to life change—because they are afraid of the body count. Go back to the notes and lists you have made about all the changes you want to make and link it to the body count. Write down all of your dreams, ranging from the outlandish to the ordinary. Which of your aspirations and changes do you believe (correctly or incorrectly— you don't know yet) would result in losses, and who would you lose? Could you tolerate that loss?

In this final exercise, build upon the dreams and associated body counts. If you believe you would lose the love or esteem of your grandmother if you got divorced, then write her a letter expressing your feelings (don't make it an e-mail —it's too easy to mistakenly and prematurely hit "send"). You do not have to send it; in fact, she may never see it. But writing down those feelings can help you sort them out, face those fears, and possibly open a conversation with that person. You may also choose to send it, but always let it breathe for a bit and then do what feels right. At a minimum, when you can see the connection between holding back on anything and the potential body count, it can help you understand the barriers you face.

CHECK-IN: BODY COUNT

Where will the bodies fall when you make life's big moves? Envision that. Think about how your choices will affect the people around you, and picture what the landscape of your life will look like on the other side of your changes. How does that feel? Can you live with it? Weigh out the difference between not doing what you want for you versus saving someone else's feelings. How often does avoiding a body count lead you to avoid your own spider senses?

CHAPTER 17

The Mindful Moment

What we think, we become . . .

—Buddha

I had the privilege of traveling through Tibet a few years ago. During my journey, I would occasionally see meditation huts high up on mountaintops. The air was so thin throughout the country that flights of stairs were an aerobic wake-up call. I couldn't imagine getting up to those huts. Yet monks would climb to those sparse and cold spaces and spend days and weeks in meditation. This was definitely hard-core.

The way most of us think about (and can actually engage in) meditation is a little different than what I witnessed in Tibet. Frankly, most of us think meditation sounds boring. Meditation is just a reboot. It's a moment (or moments) when we stop and power down, and let our minds clear out—a bit like whisking a feather duster over the bits of junk that clog our brain and our spider senses. (For most people, it would be nothing short of transcendent for them to simply switch off the devices and unwire for a few minutes.)

But meditation doesn't have to be all chanting, yoga mats, and New Age mantras. I was raised on this practice, so I come at it from a different perspective, but I can see how people may find the way it is done in the West a bit affected and cloying. Somehow my mother, grandmothers, aunts, and many others managed to build it into the day. Wherever it is done, meditation is about quieting the mind, even if just for a few minutes. It can be done on the subway in the morning, or in your bedroom in the evening. Trust me; I know it takes time and effort to really still the brain.

MEDITATION CAN CHANGE YOUR BRAIN

For a long time we believed that the brain stopped changing in adulthood—that the brain growth observed in childhood eventually ends. Mounting evidence suggests otherwise, and cutting-edge

Meditation is just a reboot. It's a moment (or moments) when we stop and power down, and let our minds clear out—a bit like whisking a feather duster over the bits of junk that clog our brain and our spider senses.

work on awareness shows that mindfulness practices, such as those used in meditation, can lead to real changes in brain structure and function. Simply put, throughout our lives, how we think, how we talk, and how we love actually shapes our brains.

Interestingly, our brains are wired for negativity—and that makes sense. Brains needed to be wired to sense danger in order for us to stay alive and evolve. Perhaps there are no longer saber-toothed tigers lurking around corners, but our brains haven't changed much, and as such we do hold on to negative memories with more strength than positive ones. Our minds sometimes want a break, and things like denial, numbing, and distraction are ways of avoiding uncomfortable feelings or other demands. The problem is that this numbing also silences our spider senses, making us less able to identify what we are feeling and how it affects our behavior. We can train our minds to focus on the positive, to welcome feelings—good and bad—but that requires us to stop, pay attention, and make a concerted effort to turn our minds in that direction.

Numerous authors, including Rick Hanson and Rich Mendius, the authors of a wonderful book called *Buddha's Brain: The Practical Neuroscience of Happiness,* write about how we can harness mindfulness and work on staying in the moment to create not only real changes in our brains, but also in our lives. Mindfulness is quite simply concentration—the ability to focus on the now and shut out the rest. You've heard the term *Be present,* right? That's the now. Our brains are socially responsive organs, wired to integrate the feedback of the outer world. By adopting elements of meditative practices, we can get in better touch with our spider senses, quiet the noise each day, and stay true to ourselves. Instead of feeding yourself with food you aren't really hungry for, feed yourself with a bit of stillness.

I can already see you rolling your eyes. Give it a chance. At worst it is just a moment of relaxation, and the potential benefits are quite amazing. Our brains actually benefit from mindfulness—that's what I want you to take away from this discussion. We learn by paying attention to things, and we can decide what to pay attention to (or to be mindful of). We have already established that we can help ourselves through those rough patches in the day when we are depleted and have less willpower just by paying attention. You can also choose whether to focus on the good or the bad. That's your choice. Basically, to put it in second-grade-speak, "You are the boss of your brain." You can try simple things like taking difficult days and pairing them with wonderful experiences and choices.

Hanson and Mendius make the excellent point that the brain constructs reality almost like a visual simulation machine, to run mini movies. At times it makes sense for us to replay these little movies. They might help us to rehearse dangers and consider possible future scenarios. That's great as a strategy for dealing with dangers in the environment, such as insects, animals, or other threats. We also use these little movies as mental shortcuts—solutions that we craft on the basis of what we think will happen.

Unfortunately, we often spend more time in the multiplex of our mind instead of staying in real life, replaying everything over and over, or watching a movie that won't be airing in our life for weeks, or scripting out the life we want instead of actually living it. Scripts can be useful as ways of managing some dangers, but the real danger of these mini movies is that we stop living in the moment and try to outguess the future. Often these mini movies are vulnerable to the usual spider-sense threats, such as fears and stakeholders. This results in our living lives that are disconnected from the moment.

When we take all of the evidence on why we eat and how we eat, and ultimately, why we live and how we live, it boils down to a few simple truths:

- In general, *our bodies do tell us what we need to know,* and we have the power to act on it. These are our spider senses—they give us a road map, but then we need to cast off the restrictions we place on ourselves and act on them.

- *By using our minds, and simply paying attention,* by avoiding the blindness and retaining focus—and as such, allowing our spider senses in—we can walk away from second helpings, from toxic relationships, and from other negative behaviors.

- This is not about prepackaged meals or prepackaged lives. This is about *listening to your own life and taking responsibility for it,* whether it's for the piece of cake that goes into your mouth or the broken marriage you decided to endure.

BEING MINDFUL EVERYWHERE

Mindfulness is the best tool we have to manage lapses in willpower, temptation, and all the nasty influences on our spider senses. Mindfulness allows us to turn down the volume button that lets in the voices from the outside and draws our attention away from what we need to do. When you eat, pay attention to the eating, which means slowing down. Mindfulness has myriad other benefits as well. It helps us worry less, reduces stress, regulates our emotions, may benefit memory, helps us stay focused when we are upset, and is even associated with more satisfaction in our relationships (Davis & Hayes, 2011).

If the idea of learning to be mindful overwhelms you, fear not. There are mindfulness practices I'm going to offer you to help calibrate yourself, and they can be built into your daily routine. Just remember to stay honest with yourself, identifying the things that may interfere with your finely honed spider senses, and learning how to apply them to life and how you eat. Everyone's meditative practice will be different. I was raised in a Hindu family where meditation was a part of our religious rituals and my mother's day-to-day routine, but it slipped away from me after I moved out. It is through the practice of accessible meditative practices that I was able to connect back with my spider senses again. The goal here is to learn to quiet the outside voices, listen to the self, and rewire your gut instincts.

The mind can be trained—this we know—but we all need to find different spaces in which to adjust and train our own. Remember the reason for this meditative practice: to help you think about the future you want by learning to listen to yourself in the present moment. This may mean that you'll have to face the changes that need to be made and accept the fears of things not turning out the way you want. Whether you jump off from this book and actually start building meditative practices into your daily life, or you just walk away committed to things like the mindfulness minute at times when you feel depleted, mindfulness and meditation are great ways to stop the noise and allow your spider senses a chance to shine through.

The following places or activities can enhance mindfulness:

- a quiet place outside,

- exercising, even taking a long, slow walk,

- listening to music that is either evocative or calming, and/or

- a room that's available to you that feels peaceful.

It's important to simply slow down. Talk slower, eat slower, live slower. Everything on your to-do list will get done, and in fact, I'd argue, you will be more efficient. Eating slower may be one of the simplest tips for eating less. It gives your mind a chance to catch up, and it gives you the opportunity to stop and be with your food. Eating quickly often leads to eating blindly.

Mindfulness is also about paying attention. Much of this book is about being aware so you can hear your spider senses when they talk to you, and also about being conscious of the influence of fears, stakeholders, and golden rules. Remember when we talked about willpower? Baumeister notes that paying attention is our best tool against lapses in willpower. When we are aware, we are better at monitoring. Attention can also be quite useful in gatekeeping—whether it's how much food goes on your plate, how much you eat, or signs at the beginning of a relationship that something's not right. We are often so distracted that we miss the data that's right in front of us. Remember what we said about the scientific method? Data is good, as long as we can integrate it while listening to ourselves. Mindfulness allows you to be the best possible scientist, and it allows data in to co-exist with your spider senses.

Attention is the key to mindfulness, and we can train our minds. We can build up our attentional capacities the same way we build muscle in the gym. Focus on a single task at a time, breathe while you do it, and keep bringing your focus back to that task. Over time you will see that you obtain better results, do better work, and make better decisions when you retain that mindful focus.

I have included check-ins throughout this book—no writing, no doing, just thinking. Mindfulness and mindful moments are not just about clearing your mind; they are also about waiting that one beat before eating, speaking, or acting. A moment to let your spider senses have a say in the noisy arcade of stakeholders, fears, and golden rules. You have already been engaging in mindful moments by engaging in the check-ins. Now you are ready to build mindfulness into your life. Stop starving yourself and mindlessly exercising. It's time to use your mind—the organ that was the main contributor to these eating, living, and loving issues—as a tool to get your health and your life back.

THE WHY

Welcome to the present. This is where you want your mind to be; this is where you want to live. The amount of time wasted on the past is the equivalent of burning money. The past is like a mine of precious metals embedded in worthless rock; once the lessons are extracted from the past, there is little left there that's of any use to you at all. The key to meditative practices is to stay in the moment. But to do this in a balanced manner, you need to remember that self-regulation is a dance between taking the long view—how a choice today can affect you down the road—and staying present. If you are able to self-monitor and remain mindful, you will be much more likely to listen to your spider senses, which generally allow for that balance to occur.

THE NOW

When you meditate, especially initially, you will be distracted by other images cycling through your mind. Invite them in; don't fight them. Just like most things in life, when you meditate, those thoughts will pass on through and have less power over time as you get better at paying attention.

Guess what will happen next? You'll be true to you. Imagine if you treated yourself the way you deserve to be treated? Imagine if you eliminated the self-doubt, self-hatred, and self-destructive thoughts that you have as your own worst critic and your worst enemy? We eat, drink, drug, shop, and do many other things to fill the emptiness left behind by those terrible thoughts and behaviors. Most of us were not born into a world of empathy and unconditional love, so to fill that hole, we do things that are at best temporary fixes, which will harm us in the long term. Here's what I propose instead:

Don't sweat not having the best start in life, or the hurts you have suffered; give it to yourself now.

Do not wait to be rescued; *rescue yourself.*

Treat yourself well. Celebrate yourself; look for the good in you and celebrate it. Find opportunities to do this every day.

Live. The more actively you live your life, the less you will eat or engage in other exercises in blind "filling." You will uncover your spider senses, because when you like yourself you will trust yourself. Healthier eating and activity is such a great example of this. Initially, weight management involves putting healthier things into your body, using your body, and paying attention to what you eat and what you do. Over time, as you no longer numb yourself with extra weight and food, your spider senses will start running more openly, and you'll establish a cycle whereby you are taking better care of yourself. Weight loss often precedes our ability to advocate for ourselves, fight for ourselves, and ultimately, love ourselves.

Voice your intention. Visualize your intention. Live your intention. You will then find yourself living in that direction and subtly and before you know it, you will be doing it. Instead of spending your time mired in regret about what you didn't do, spend it thinking about what you want to do. Then just do it.

Build your breathing into life. Just like you wash your hands before eating, breathe before and while doing the stuff of life. It will make you more mindful while you are engaged in a task. Your brain needs oxygen just like it needs food. Feed it by breathing deeply. Pay attention to your breath, and break it down—focus on the inhale, on how it feels; focus on the exhale, and count if you have to.

Stop multitasking. Our brains were not made for this. You may think you are multitasking, but in fact you are multifailing. Efficiency and accuracy decrease, and you become depleted and more likely to succumb to lapses in regulation and willpower. Electronics and devices trick us into thinking we can do it all, but in reality, they just give us new ways of making mistakes and pulling us out of the moment.

Unwire once a day. Once a day put down the smartphone and shut down. Unless you are on call for emergency services, try to unplug for ten to fifteen minutes a day, preferably more. Not talking, texting, surfing, or playing Words with Friends will allow mindfulness to grow, and your spider senses will sharpen as a result.

Practice infectious calmness. Most things you get excited about are not worth it, so remain calm. If you do, more calm will follow, and all will be well. Most situations are manageable if you keep a cool head.

Practice gratitude. Once a day, find a way to reflect on an experience, person, or event that has filled you with gratitude. By staying on the lookout for it, you will generate more and more gratitude, whether you're giving or receiving it. This is a far better way of meeting your needs than stuffing them with food.

Share mindfulness. In a relationship, take a moment to look into the face and eyes of your partner and just pay attention to the feelings you have. Some practitioners even suggest that while looking at your partner, you quietly share and send good loving feelings to the other.

Break down the meal. Sometimes mindful eating can be a challenge for folks who have been eating mindlessly for a long time. While eating, break down the meal in your mind. "Smelling food, sticking fork into food, lifting fork, placing food in mouth, tasting garlic, chewing slowly, swallowing . . ." This may seemed hackneyed, but do it every so often as a way to slow down and, more mindfully, eat less food.

Eat slowly. Mindful-eating experts suggest that you literally think about where the food came from—how it was grown, harvested, and brought to your table. By doing that at each step, and chewing slowly, the meal will become a place of mindfulness and more satisfaction. The exercise below will help you with that.

Sleep. Sleep. Sleep. Most of us don't get enough rest. Mindfulness requires a rested mind, and we are more likely to have lapses in willpower and difficulties with listening to our inner voices and spider senses when we are fatigued. I actually think sleep may be a more useful weight-loss tool than exercise.

Mindful-Eating Exercise

I am guessing that for many of you, your last meal may have involved wolfing down a burger while at a red light, or even eating something healthy at a red light. It's time to invite your mind to the table, whether it's breakfast, dinner, or just a snack. Here is an exercise that will help you begin to eat more mindfully:

1. Set the table. This means plate, utensils, napkin, flowers—even a candle. Make it a pleasant experience. If you eat lunch at work, set out a paper napkin and plastic fork, your water, and if possible, enjoy your food anywhere other than at your desk.

2. Put food you like in front of you in a proper portion size.

3. Eat, and only eat. Do not read, watch TV, or do anything else.

4. Cut your food slowly and pay attention to the smells, tastes, and sounds.

5. Chew each bite slowly and check in with yourself after each bite.

I recognize that most meals cannot be consumed this way, but it's a way of feeling and experiencing what eating more slowly and ceremoniously feels like. Even that burger at the stoplight can be eaten more slowly, by taking smaller bites, enjoying longer chewing time, and thinking about each bite as you chew it.

In general I would suggest that you stop eating on the fly. How often do you eat your dinner over the sink, a sandwich in the car, or a meal in a meeting? Sometimes we do this out of necessity, and believe me when I say, living in Los Angeles with our epic traffic, I am more guilty of this than anyone. But in such settings we make many mistakes. Eating at a stoplight or while doing anything else is the absolute polar opposite of mindful eating. Driving demands our full attention, which means we are less mindful when we eat in such settings.

We tend to rush, and since our attention is being pulled to a demanding activity (driving in traffic), we have less attention to monitor our eating. Eating fast often leads us to eat too much—just like living fast makes us miss the good stuff. We are often in such a rush to get to the next thing that we miss the beauty of what is right in front of us.

Here are a few other tips that will help you eat with more ceremony and more mindfulness:

- *Turn every meal at home into a special occasion,* the way you feel at a restaurant. Put out candles and flowers, and set the table. Make it a presentation. This can slow you down.

- Even if you're alone, *set a place at your kitchen or dining room table,* not your coffee table in front of the couch.

- Fill your plate in the kitchen, put the food away, and *sit and eat only what is on the plate.*

- *Eat without distractions.* I have the bad habit of reading while I eat, and I know that many people watch TV during their meals. The problem again is that we let the environment set the pace of the meal, making us unable to monitor our eating or spider senses. (I keep eating until the chapter is done; some people get up and eat more during the commercials or when the action on the show slows down.)

- Talk while you eat so that you eat more slowly. One tool that works well for me, when my daughters are at their father's home for a week or weekend and I'm alone, is that if I do need to eat by myself, I sometimes make a phone call during the meal and put the phone on speaker, because the fits and stops of conversation mean that I sometimes need to stop eating in order to have my conversation (I try not to eat crunchy things during these chats!). It slows me down and lets satiety kick in.

The Daily-Doubt Diary and Purge

Let's be done with doubting ourselves! Done. Finished. Who wants to think about doubts at the end of the day?

Many different sources can enhance self-doubt. We have friends who look askance at our decisions. Our boss may discourage our ideas at work, deflating our excitement. When we doubt, we make mistakes. Fear also drives self-doubt.

Instead, let's reflect on those doubts each day in an effort to allow our spider senses to get back up to speed. How? I actually keep a doubt diary, and I propose you do the same. I have an alarm set on my cell phone which goes off around 7:30 p.m. At that point each day I reflect on something that I second-guessed, or felt second-guessed on. It will often help my spider senses recalibrate, remind me of what I want, who I want to be, and what I am willing to give up. It's easy to plow through the day blindly, and oddly, my doubtful meditation moment each day actually often brings a sharper focus and allows me to be less hard on myself.

To get maximal utility out of this exercise, you should write it down each day—the doubt you have, and the reflection brought in when your alarm sounded. The accumulation of data will show you where doubt gets inserted, and who or what inserts it. It will also keep you focused on the things that you are willing to fight for. (Think about times when your stakeholders asked, "Are you sure?") Otherwise, the doubt can start to accumulate like fat around your midsection, and if you wait too long, it's very hard to eliminate.

By completing this exercise, you'll get rid of doubt once a day. You can view this doubtful meditation exercise as a bit of a "fat-burner" for your soul.

The Five-Minute Fix

Remove yourself from the world. Lock yourself in the bathroom or closet if you must. Set a timer for five minutes.

Just sit. Don't feel like you need to do some aspirational "empty your mind" thing, but also, don't read, don't watch TV, and turn off your phone.

Close your eyes if you want, or keep them open.

Breathe. Breathe in slowly, through your nose. Hold it, and then exhale slowly through your nose. Most of the time we breathe too shallowly, making us feel like we're on the brink of hyperventilating all day. Over time you will start emptying your mind without even thinking about it.

Think of all the little five-minute bits you waste in a day. All you need to do is sit and breathe. Don't pressure yourself to be some sort of Zen guru; just let go through your breath. Mix it up if you like, and do your breathing in different places. Every so often, do it in a beautiful place like at the beach, in the forest, or in a park. If all you have is the subway, close your eyes and breathe there. Or sit in your parked car, at your desk, on a plane, or on a bus, and breathe deeply.

CHECK-IN: MINDFULNESS

Once you've done five minutes a day, think about how differently you react to things. Does it help? Can you mentally note if you moved differently or in a different direction as a result? For this check-in, I just want you to assess the effectiveness of meditation and being mindful. Try out some different things. Some people try to clear their minds; some welcome in the noise around them and let it fill them like white noise. Just like no one else can tell you how to eat, no one can tell you how to meditate and find that quiet place in your mind.

CHAPTER 18

Anarchy or Authenticity?

Know the rules well, so you can break them effectively.
—Dalai Lama XIV

I have something to add to the Dalai Lama's words: ". . . and know your-self so you can break them wisely."

You're empowered now that you've come this far in the book. You have the tools to think and live differently. These are the first steps to being authentic in your life: listening to your spider senses, and being true to yourself as you reflect on what you want your life to look like. One of the main criticisms I hear about trusting your gut and doing what you feel is right for you is this: "If everyone did whatever they felt like doing, wouldn't society fall apart?"

Quite the contrary, I believe. We have become so skilled at denying our instinctual nature that we have developed all kinds of ugly defenses in response to it. For example, how often do we see politicians spouting off about morality and then discover them in compromising positions? Think of it this way: Life becomes an internal game of "Whack-a-mole." If you deny something, it will just pop out someplace else, and usually in a less-healthy form. We often deprive ourselves of food only to ultimately give up and start eating in an out-of-control manner. That's why we have so much yo-yo dieting in this country. People starve themselves to lose weight, but then gain even more back when they resume eating from all the food groups, and then some. That's a huge contributor to weight gain nationwide, the varying between excessive control and dyscontrol. The actual anarchy comes when we deny our authentic sense of knowing what our bodies need in terms of food, activity, and satiety. Anarchy would ensue if we stopped listening to our spider senses completely.

It likely has happened to your body at some point, but I'd rather it not happen to you again. By not listening to yourself and your body, you don't know how to feed it, so you may eat blindly, spend blindly, or live blindly. And that may have thrown your own life into unlawful disorder, while the world around you remained orderly. It's time to change that.

> *The actual anarchy comes when we deny our authentic sense of knowing what our bodies need in terms of food, activity, and satiety. Anarchy would ensue if we stopped listening to our spider senses.*

FINDING AUTHENTICITY

> *At the center of your being*
> *you have the answer;*
> *you know who you are*
> *and you know what you want.*
> —Lao Tzu

We overuse the word *authentic*. In my simple lexicon it means "keeping it real." It doesn't mean living a script, but rather living a real life. Now, to do that, you need to own up to the very characteristics that make you, you, even if they don't fall in line with what's expected. Live your script, not the one provided by the world around you.

As I say this, I know it's not easy. We often compromise with some "soft-scripted" lives, partly doing what we want and partly doing what's expected. We think we are doing our own thing, but we are actually obediently living the scripts fed to us by the world (just like the plates of food they give us), and we have been doing it for so long that we start to believe that they are our own.

Here's a great way to start living this authentic life and not caving to the majority opinion: Instead of wondering, "What's wrong with me?" when you don't live the way everyone else around you is living, say to yourself, "This is me." Change the conversation; alter the dialogue—that's the first step to authenticity. And always, always remember, authenticity need not be an act of defiance. It can be soft, organic, and quiet. There's no need to defend ourselves when we buck the trends. Defending yourself wastes tremendous psychological resources. Just be.

Authenticity is about listening to yourself and being mindful. When you feel that you're not dancing to the music of others, if you're authentic, you will be less angry and resentful, and less likely to behave in ways that don't make sense to you. I believe and have witnessed through my years of clinical work and teaching—and most important, living—that those who live in a more authentic way emanate tremendous kindness, little jealousy, and lots of unconditional support. Because their lives are about honoring themselves, it extends outward, and they give that gift of authenticity to others, rarely judging, always supporting. In fact, these folks that are likely viewed as authentic anarchists are generally more ethical and rule-abiding than their script-following counterparts.

FEAR OF AUTHENTICITY

It is fear that lives deep in the mind-set of the nonbelievers, the script followers, and the people who love social order. The fear is that if everyone lived authentically, then no one would ever get married or commit to anything. I disagree. Not only do I believe people would commit, I think for once they would succeed. They would commit to something from a place of want, and see it through with genuineness rather than a forced sense of obligation. If they commit from an authentic space rather than from a fictional one, they will be in line with their spider senses, with themselves, and that commitment to self will translate to commitment to what they believe in: partnership, parenting, work, school.

Recently, I had a conversation with someone about a relationship I am in, and the person asked me, "What will you do if he hurts you?" In the past I would have played it cool, and would have rarely confessed to the depth of feelings I had for a man, believing that if I did, I would be hurt even more. But the feelings were real, I was having them, and my not acknowledging them didn't make them less real. In fact, I was creating a fiction by not being honest, and so while I appeared like a cool customer to the world, almost indifferent, inside I was not, and when it fell apart (which it typically did), I would fall apart, too.

This time I own it. It is a complex relationship. I am deeply in love, he has the power to hurt me, and if he betrayed me or left me, I would experience true painful loss. But right now he is a source of tremendous joy, so I scream his name from the rooftops. I tell my friends I am in love. My friends tell me they are "protecting me." But right now, today, it is real, and so in line with that, I speak about it and live it as such. If a day dawns where he hurts me, that won't change the joy we have had; instead of looking back at me holding back, I will know that I gave it my all, was witness to something beautiful, and because of that openness, I'll likely find such joy again. To hold back today in the name of an unnamed future is not real, and would hold me back from the full joy of this experience. Perhaps the strength I get now will give me the strength I need down the road. We purchase insurance to cover our butts in a variety of situations, but there is nothing like that in life, and caution does not purchase safety. Take a moment to enjoy what you have today, because you cannot hoard happiness; it is something that must be consumed in the moment.

THE WHY

I encourage you to really listen to you and to live an authentic life. There is no insurance policy on life, but if you live an authentic life, own it all, you'll find happiness, you'll find success, you'll achieve weight loss, and you'll empower yourself. There's simply no other way.

THE NOW

Now you're armed. I've asked you to complete a lot of different exercises throughout this book, really thinking about your life. But this is different, because now you understand the pillars of my theory: stakeholders, gate-keeping, fear, fables and fairy tales, and spider senses—and you're free to keep it real and envision an authentic life for yourself.

So in this exercise, answer these three questions in your journal:

- Who do you want to be?
- What do you want your life to look like?
- How much closer are you now than when you started this process?

Keep using the Promise of One. I'm guessing that some of the things you started when you first began doing the exercises may already be habits, and some changes are already occurring. Every day, keep that promise, and keep that running log.

————◄◦►————

I want to share with you my experience doing this exercise, so you'll understand that I'm where you are. I'm working through this with you.

When I conceived of this exercise I was in the midst of a waking dream. I wrote the draft of it while sitting in a cafe at the end of a dock in a little village in Italy. I had envisioned this setting months before (despite having never been here)—the backdrop, the town, the light, and the water. I saw myself as the traveling doctor, with her backpack and laptop, writing her book in various corners of the world.

And then it happened. I used the Promise of One to get here. An e-mail about the village, an exploration of plane fares, a little timing, a bit of debt, a leap of courage. The data told me it wasn't a good financial decision; my spider senses told me it was essential. And I found myself in the scene I'd envisioned.

I did the same in my career: I wanted to make an impact on the media, to share my vision and experience with the masses, and, well, here it is!

I said it out loud, and I received a few guffaws—both about the Italy trip and the media career. Now people smile and are happy for me. It awakened dreams inside those around me. I have friends who are now writing, friends who are now traveling, friends who are now starting new jobs, friends who are now leaving dead relationships, and friends who are taking a chance on love. I never told them to do it; I just lived. Authentically. You will have the same effect on others if you do this as well.

Live Your Story

Make a list of what you want your life to look like—some examples include:

- Where do you want to live?
- What do you want to do?
- What do you want for your children?
- What do you want from your relationship?
- How do you dress?
- How do you live?

This is personal, so keep it real. I am hoping that by this time in the book you are feeling braver. It could be "I want to open a bar" or "I want to write a novel." Maybe you are saying, "I want to make a documentary about my grandmother" or "I want to travel with my children," or even, "I want to run a marathon." The world is a place of infinite possibilities. You might want to climb a mountain, become a chef, or build a house. Don't be afraid to even say, "I want to fall in love." That's okay, too. Just own it.

This is not a book to read just once; it's a workbook, and one that you can tailor to your own needs. Circle back, reflect on your answers, look at the changes over time, add to it, and subtract (maybe you try something out and your spider senses tell you it isn't working for you). Monitor your changes. Stay mindful, and harness your mind instead of viewing it as your adversary; work cooperatively and take good care of it—feed it, exercise it, and remember how it works.

Little by little, through thoughts, or through saying it aloud, release the story of your life to the world. Don't be afraid. Ironically, as I write these final words, I am in New York City, about twenty-three blocks and twenty-three years from where this journey began, when I started my training as a psychologist. Lots of spider senses got silenced, lots of stakeholders weighed in, lots of fears were fought, lots of golden rules were broken, and there was more than a small body count. Twenty-three years of the Promise of One. This is not about weight loss for an event; it's about weight loss for life. This is not about thinking of making a few changes; this is about living the life you want.

CHECK-IN: AUTHENTICITY

To me, it was once laughable that I would find myself in Italy and subsequently New York, finishing up this book. Here I am. I drowned out the voices. I went for it. I listened to me. But first I had to figure out what that would look like. That is what I hope for you. Make this check-in a promise to yourself. Honor yourself and live authentically. I hope each day for you ends with the same joy, the same sense of accomplishment, and the same feeling of empowerment that comes with the journey. And remember to keep checking back in with yourself—what you want for yourself today is different from what you may want tomorrow. Give yourself room to try new things, and to walk away from things that no longer feel right.

Who do you want to be?

Become it.

EPILOGUE

I'm happy to say that this book has a happy ending.

I recently began speaking about the principles in this book. At one event I found myself in front of an audience of undergraduate students and giving them the broad ideas. A woman with whom I work stood up and said, "Let me really tell you what this book is about." I was a bit surprised, but I gave her the floor.

This woman is part of the staff of my lab and has been observing me working for years, both early mornings and late nights, through frantic deadlines and a few bouts of paralytic anxiety. I tried to squeeze writing in between all of my other responsibilities, and I wasn't sure my staff was aware of my bizarre balancing act. But on this day she stood in front of the group and said, "Dr. Ramani Durvasula has been working on this book and living the words every day I have known her. She talks about it regularly. It's not just a book. About a year ago I started paying attention and trying to put into practice what she was saying. One thing a day." I thought that was nice and was about to start speaking again when she kept going.

She floored me with what followed. She went on to say that in the last year she had lost sixty pounds. She had reached out to a long-ago love and gotten married. She was inspired to take on new direction in her work, blending her interests in diabetes and HIV. Most amazingly, she said she had learned to listen to herself and throw away all the bad diet advice she had received over the years. She said, "I don't just have a new body; I have a new life." It was moving for me to hear her say that she'd done it, after all of these years, with the help of my book. She capped it off by saying that for the first time in a decade, she no longer had to take medications to manage her diabetes.

She made it sound simple because it *is* simple. She listened to herself, took on her stakeholders, tolerated the body count, and carved out a new path for her life by doing just one thing a day.

It's not just her. Since then, others who have been reading early versions of this book are sharing with me successful tales of weight lost, love found, lives rebuilt, dreams attempted, screenplays written, trips taken, paintings sold—and most important, tales of finally putting down the scripts and listening to themselves.

Her story alone makes this entire book worth it to me: one life changed. I hope that whatever journey this book takes you on, it leads you home to you.

ACKNOWLEDGMENTS

This book is not just an opportunity to share clinical and research wisdom, it is also a life story and a love story. Although my name is on it, it is actually a collaboration of a glorious cast of courageous characters who believed in me, shared their stories, and encouraged me to put it down on paper.

To each of you who were willing to take a chance on a new-comer—you trusted your spider senses (I hope). My literary agent Maura Teitelbaum, manager Tanya Hekimian-Brogan, and agent Mark Turner. With tremendous gratitude to Lara Asher and everyone at Globe Pequot Press (and to Ellen for taking this on line by line), and especially to you Stephanie Krikorian. Lara and Stephanie, your editorial patience and friendship have been sublime even as I become verbose and incomprehensible. I look forward to some down time with both of you soon.

To my teachers, who cultivated in me the love of literature, writing, science, philosophy, psychology, poetry, and music. With special gratitude to Dr. Hector Myers and Dr. Eric Miller for never letting me give up on my vision.

To my students, who have been my teachers as well and push me to learn more every day.

To my patients—I am privileged to have been allowed into your private space. Each of you is courageous for taking on the journey of growth and actualization.

To the thousands of research participants I have worked with, especially in the world of HIV. Your candor and bravery have been stunning, and though you don't always realize it, you have changed the world with your openness.

To my friends, my unconditional stakeholders, who never let me stop dreaming, kept me on deadline, and pushed me to keep at it even when I didn't have the fight anymore. Jill Davenport, Kara Sullivan, Christine Anderson, Mona Baird, Debbie Raisner, Tonia Mendinghall, Eric Miller, Eric Borsum, Fary Cachelin, Seth Meyer, Stephanny Freeman, Munyi Shea, Tammi Fuller, Bryan Donovan, Miguel Rossy, Dee Lewis, Efren Briseno, Kathi Mead, Kieran Sullivan, Pamela Regan, Cheryl Johnson, Mara Silverman, Tasnim Shamji, Toni Lewis, Shellye Jones, Greg Lyon, and to

Emily Shagley, for lighting enough candles to bring down a forest. I love you all, so very much. Bless you for keeping me standing when I couldn't.

To my friends who had the task of making me presentable—Shay Bacher, Dan Musto, Stacey Rosas, Travis Walters, Dolores Montero, Paige Craig, and Sonia Jimenez. Thank you for your friendship and for overhauling my outsides on a dime. You worked with an impossible candidate and you made me beautiful inside and out.

To Morgan Wilson, for loving my daughters when I could not be there. This would have been impossible without you and I am grateful you are part of our funny little family.

To Dr. Pamela Harmell—in many respects this journey started with you. I hate to say it, but you were my salvation.

To my research team at California State University Los Angeles—Orenda Warren, Daisy De Jesus-Sosa, Kimberlee Chronister, Judy Lam-Tran, Karen Keen, and Alex Indaco, and to my research teams from the past many years. You have patiently supported my dreams and our lab, and had my back.

To the colleagues I have worked with through my governance work at the American Psychological Association and through the Leadership Institute for Women in Psychology—thank you for forcing me to articulate my dream of writing a book. With special thanks to Drs. Steven Brady, Perry Halkitis, Scyatta Wallace, Sandy Schullman, David Tolin, John Anderson, and Norman Anderson.

To the folks at California State University, Los Angeles, for giving me an academic home to pursue my scholarship and teaching.

To the many wonderful producers and crew members I have worked with in the TV world—Jeff, Roy, Jenn, Robbie, Angie, Wendy, Emily, Michaline, and Esther. You taught me how to get to the point, how to smile, where to look, and how to keep it sharp and simple. And especially to Dr. Drew Pinsky for being a mentor as I entered the realm of media mental health; you taught me the delicate balance of clinical science and TV. I look forward to continuing our collaborations.

To the myriad people I have met on my travels as I wrote this book for a smile, a shared coffee, for pulling up a chair when you saw me sitting alone, and for your beautiful stories. A special gratitude to Sandro Levi and the people of Lerici, Italy, where I wrote some of the richest sections of this book. I will be back soon . . .

To Hitomi Uchishiba, for every broken heart you eased me through. And for the tea and sunrise on Mt. Fuji.

To Robert Mack—you changed my landscape and introduced me to myself. There are no words.

To Vanessa Williams, for your foreword, your friendship, and your faith in me.

To Charlie Hinkin, with you I share the greatest gift—our children. I am grateful to have shared a marriage with you and to watch our children grow up together. Thank you for your friendship and for being an extraordinary father.

To my parents, Rao and Sai Durvasula—we continue on a complex journey together. I understand all you sacrificed to make a life possible in which I have the freedom to honor myself. Love is challenging, but it is still love. Thank you.

To Padma, Joe, and Tanner Salisbury for the joy, and Padma for the secret space, laughter, and language we have always shared.

To Bill Pruitt—you, my love, are a wonder. I gave up the ship on love and then you came sailing in. I look forward to a lifetime of poetry, mysticism, sunrises, moonsets, mountaintops, and editing each other's words.

To Maya and Shanti Hinkin—this book is for you. My voice forever telling you to honor your hearts, listen to yourselves, take chances, and be brave. These pages represent your sacrifice, time away from you, performances missed, bad dinners, late nights, and early mornings. You are my inspiration in everything I do. With each of your births, my spider senses came alive. I love you.

NOTES

INTRODUCTION

Kabir (Indian mystic 1440–1518), "The Simple Purification," *The Forty-Four Ecstatic Poems of Kabir.*

For more information on Simon Rodia and Watts Towers:

Bud Goldstone, Arloa Goldstone, and Arloa Paquin Goldstone. *The Los Angeles Watts Towers* (Getty Conservation Institute, 1997).

How Americans Eat Today. CBS News and *USA Today.* January 12, 2010, hyperlink: cbsnews.com/2100-500165_162-6086647.html.

F. Le Duc de la Rochefoucauld (Brown, E. translation), *Maxims* (1917).

CHAPTER 1

Lao Tzu, *Tao Te Ching* (J. Legge translation).

Henry Miller, *Henry Miller on Writing* (1964).

Amazing Spider-Man #1, Stan Lee, ed. (1963).

Michael Gershon, *The Second Brain: A Groundbreaking New Understanding of Nervous Disorders of the Stomach and Intestine* (Harper Perennial, 1999).

Antoine Bechara, and Antonio R. Damasio, "The somatic marker hypothesis: A neural theory of economic decision," *Games and Economic Behavior,* vol. 52 (2005): 336–72.

Antoine Bechara, Hanna Damasio, and Antonio R. Damasio, "Emotion, decision making, and the orbitofrontal cortex," *Cerebral Cortex* (2000), 295–307.

Sigmund Freud, *Civilization and Its Discontents* (1930).

CHAPTER 2

Lao Tzu, *Tao Te Ching* (J. Legge translation).

Stanleu Milgram, *Obedience to Authority: An Experimental View* (Harper Collins, 1974).

Edith Wharton, *The Age of Innocence* (first published in 1920, Barnes and Noble Classics, 2004) 288.

Marjorie Garber, and Nancy J. Vickers, eds., *The Medusa Reader* (Routledge, 2003).

Charles Bukowski, *Tales of Ordinary Madness* (1967).

CHAPTER 3

George Bernard Shaw, *Maxims for Revolutionists* (1903).

Aesop's Fables (Simon and Brown, 2012).

Hans Christian Andersen, *The Red Shoes* (1845).

Ramayana (originally composed by Valmiki somehere between the 8th and 5th centuries BC). Modern translations include those by Ramesh Menon, North Point Press, 2004; and Arshia Sattar, Penguin Global, 2003).

Bruno Bettelheim, *The Uses of Enchantment: The Meaning and Importance of Fairy Tales* (1976).

Walter Isaacson, *Steve Jobs* (Simon and Schuster, 2011).

Ambrose Bierce, *The Devil's Dictionary* (1911).

Warren Buffett (unsourced).

Sleepless in Seattle, Tri-Star Pictures (1993).

T. A. Judge, "Core self-evaluations and work success," *Current Directions in Psychological Science* (2009), 18 (1): 59-62.

CHAPTER 4

Victor Frankl, *Man's Search for Meaning* (1946).

Albert Ellis, *Reason and Emotion in Psychotherapy: A Comprehensive Method of Treating Human Disturbances* (Citadel, 1994).

Ivan P. Pavlov, *Conditioned Reflexes* (Oxford, England: Oxford University Press, 1927).

Roy Baumeister, *Willpower: Rediscovering the Greatest Human Strength* (Penguin Books, 2011).

Roy Baumeister, and Kathleen Vohs, "Self-regulation, ego depletion, and motivation," *Social and Personality Psychology Compass* (2007), 1(1): 1–14.

Roy Baumiester, Kathleen Vohs, and George Loewenstein, ed., "Willpower, choice, and self-control," *Time and Decision: Economic and Psychological Perspectives on Intertemporal Choice* (Russell Sage Foundation, 2003).

Mark Muraven, "Building self-control strength: Practicing self-control leads to improved self-control performance," *Journal of Experimental and Social Psychology* (2010), vol. 46 (1):465–68.

Wilhelm Hofmann, Roy F. Baumeister, Georg Foster, and Kathleen D. Vohs, "Everyday temptations: An experience sampling study of desire, conflict, and self-control," *Journal of Personality and Social Psychology* (2012), vol. 102 (6):1318–1355.

Jean M. Twenge, and Roy F. Baumeister, "Self control: A limited yet renewable resource," *Self and Identity: Personal, Social & Symbolic* (edited by Y. Kashima, M. Foddy, and M. Platow, Psychology Press, 2002).
Like Crazy (Paramount Vantage and Indian Paintbrush, 2011).

CHAPTER 5
Mark Twain, *Following the Equator: A Journey Around the World* (1897).
Antonio R. Damasio, *Descartes Error: Emotion, Reason and the Human Brain* (Harper Perennial, 1995).
Daniel Gilbert, *Stumbling on Happiness* (Knopf, 2006).

CHAPTER 6
Ralph Waldo Emerson, "Self-reliance" (essay, 1841).
Daniel Kahnemann, *Thinking, Fast and Slow* (Farrar, Straus and Giroux, 2011).
Confucius (551–479 BC), *Analects*.
Carl Jung, "Stages of life," *The Portable Jung* (edited by Joseph Campbell, translated by R.F.C. Hull, Penguin Books, original copyright 1971 for this collection).

CHAPTER 7
Vincent van Gogh (unsourced).

CHAPTER 8
Ralph Waldo Emerson (unsourced).

CHAPTER 9
Robert G. Ingersoll, *The Works of Robert G. Ingersoll* (1911).
Centers for Disease Control (2012), *National Obesity Trends,* cdc.gov/obesity/data/adult.html.
M. J. Da Silva, K. McKenzie, T. Harpham, and S. Huttley. "Social capital and mental illness: A systematic review," *Journal of Epidemiology and Community Health* (2004), 59 (8), 619–27.
S. Galea, J. Ahern, M. Tracy, S. Rudenstine, and D. Vlahov. "Education inequality and use of cigarettes, alcohol, and marijuana," *Drug and Alcohol Dependence* (2007), 90, S4–S15.

James O. Hill, Holly R. Wyatt, George W. Reed, and John C. Peters, "Obesity and the environment, where do we go from here?" *Science* (2003), vol. 299:853–55.

Xavier Pi-Sunyer, "A clinical view of the obesity problem," *Science* (2003), 299:859–60.

Katrina Kelner, and Laura Helmuth, "Obesity—What is to be done?" *Science* (2003), 299:845.

Jeffrey Friedman, "A war on obesity, not the obese," *Science* (2003), 299:856–58.

Marion Nestle, "The ironic politics of obesity," *Science* (2003), 299:799.

Rae Silver, Peter D. Balsam, Matthew P. Butler, and Joseph LeSauter, "Food anticipation depends on oscillators and memories in both body and brain," *Physiology and Behavior* (2011), vol. 104:562–71.

Marc-Andre Cornier, "Is your brain to blame for weight regain?" *Physiology and Behavior* (2011), 104:608–12.

Leann L. Birch, and Stephanie Anzman-Frasca, "Promoting children's healthy eating in obesogenic environments: Lessons learned from the rat," *Physiology and Behavior* (2011), vol. 104:641–45.

CHAPTER 10

Oscar Wilde, *The Picture of Dorian Gray* (1891).

Marshall Reid, and Alexandra Reid, *Portion Size Me* (Sourcebooks, 2012).

Roy F. Baumeister, and Jessica L. Alquist, "Is there a downside to good self-control?" *Self and Identity* (2009), Psychology Press: 115–30.

CHAPTER 11

Mark Twain (unsourced).

Portion Sizes Over Time: Centers for Disease Control.

http://hp2010.nhlbihin.net/oei_ss/PD1/slide1.htm and http://hp2010.nhlbihin.net/oei_ss/PDII/slide1.htm.

Lisa R. Young, and Marion Nestle, "The contribution of expanding portion sizes to the US obesity epidemic," *American Journal of Public Health* (2002), vol. 92(2):246–49.

Brian Wansink, James E. Painter, and Jill North, "Bottomless bowls: Why visual cues of portion size may influence intake," *Obesity Research* (2005) 13 93–100.

S. E. Swithers, and T. L. Davidson, "A role for sweet taste: Calorie predictive relations in energy regulation by rats," *Behavioral Neuroscience* (2008), 122:161–73.

S. E. Swithers, C. R. Baker, and T. L. Davidson, "General and persistent effects of high-intensity sweeteners on body weight gain and caloric compensation in rats," *Behavioral Neuroscience* (2009), 123:772–80.

Linda Bartoshuk, "Presidential column: Artificial sweeteners: Outwitting the wisdom of the body?" *APS Observer* (2009).

James A. Blumenthal, et al. "Exercise and pharmacotherapy in the treatment of major depressive disorder," *Psychosomatic Medicine* (2007), vol. 69:587–96.

Michael Otto, and Jasper A. J. Smits, *Exercise for Mood and Anxiety: Proven Strategies for Overcoming Depression and Enhancing Well-Being* (Oxford University Press, 2011).

Frank J. Penedo, and Jason R. Dahn, "Exercise and well-being: A review of mental and physical health benefits associated with physical activity," *Current Opinion in Psychiatry* (2005), vol. 18, (2):189–93.

Brenda Anderson, Daniel P. McCloskey, Nefta A. Mitchell, and Despina A. Tata, "Exercise effects on learning and neural systems," *Enhancing Cognitive Functioning and Brain Plasticity* (edited by Wotjek Chodzo-Zajko, Arthur F. Kramer, and Leonard W. Poon, Champaign, IL: Human Kinetics, 2009).

Kirsten Weir, "The exercise effect," *Monitor on Psychology* (2011), vol. 42 (11):49–52.

CHAPTER 12

Virginia Woolf, *A Room of One's Own* (1929).

CHAPTER 13

Anatole France, *Le Jardin D'Epicure* (1894).
Death Cab for Cutie, *I'll Follow You Into the Dark* (2007).
Sigmund Freud, *Civilization and Its Discontents* (1930).

CHAPTER 14

Anais Nin (unsourced).

CHAPTER 15

Kurt Vonnegut, *Slaughterhouse-Five* (1969).

K. D. Vohs, R. F. Baumeister, and N. J. Ciarocco, "Self-regulation and self-presentation: Regulatory resource depletion impairs impression management and effortful self-presentation depletes regulatory resources," *Journal of Personality and Social Psychology* (2005), 88:632–57.

K. D. Vohs, R. F. Baumeister, B. J. Schmeichel, J. M. Twenge, N. M. Nelson, and D. M. Tice, "Making choices impairs subsequent self-control: A limited resource account of decision making," *Journal of Personality and Social Psychology* (2008), 94:883–98.

K. D. Vohs, and R. J. Faber, "Spent resources: Self-regulatory resource availability affects impulse buying," *Journal of Consumer Research* (2007), 33:537–47.

K. D. Vohs, and T. F. Heatherton, "Self-regulatory failure: A resource-depletion approach." *Psychological Science* (2000), 11:249–54.

CHAPTER 16

Buddhist text (unsourced).

George Bernard Shaw, *Maxims for Revolutionists* (1903).

CHAPTER 17

Buddhist text (unsourced).

Rick Hanson and Rick Mendius, *Buddha's Brain: The Practical Neuroscience of Happiness, Love, and Wisdom* (New Harbinger Media, 2009).

D. M. Davis and J. A. Hayes. "What are the benefits of mindfulness? A practice review of psychotherapy-related research." *Psychotherapy* (2011), 48 (2), 198-208.

C. K. Germer, R. D. Siegel, and P. R. Fulton. *Mindfulness and Psychotherapy*, (Guilford Press, 2005).

CHAPTER 18

Dalai Lama XIV, *Instructions for Life*.

Lao Tzu (unsourced).

RESOURCES/TOOLS

As new resources become available, they will be made available at the website for the book: youarewhyyoueat.com.

ELLIS'S 12 IRRATIONAL BELIEFS: (ALBERT ELLIS)

1. It is a dire necessity for adults to be loved by others for almost everything they do.
2. There is the idea that certain acts are unlawful and wicked.
3. It is a horrible tragedy when things are not the way we like them to be.
4. Human misery is invariably caused by forces outside of us and is forced on us by outside people and events
5. *If something is or may be dangerous* we should be terribly upset and endlessly obsess about it.
6. It is easier to avoid than to face life difficulties and responsibilities.
7. We absolutely need something other or stronger or greater than us on which to rely.
8. We should be thoroughly competent, intelligent, and achieving in all possible respects.
9. If something once strongly affected our life, *it should indefinitely affect it.*
10. We *must* have control over things.
11. Human happiness can be achieved by inertia and inaction.
12. We have virtually no control over our emotions and cannot help feeling disturbed about things.

WEBSITES

American Psychological Association: The website of the APA offers a variety of current reports relevant to mental health and wellness, including weight management. The content is always being updated and many sections of the site are designed for the general public: apa.org.

Association for Psychological Science: The APS is an organization for research psychologists who apply science to understanding a variety of behavioral and mental health issues, and because the science is being regularly updated, recent reports related to health, weight, and wellness are frequently provided: psychologicalscience.org.

The National Institute of Mental Health has numerous layperson's fact sheets on health, mental health, mental illness, and obesity: nimh.nih.gov.

The *American Diabetes Association* provides dietary guidelines that are diabetes specific and useful for readers who are balancing the demands of weight management within the context of diabetes: diabetes.org.

Sharecare brings together expert opinion from physicians, psychologists, and other allied health professionals. (I am a contributor to this site and bring my expert opinion on a variety of health related issues.) sharecare.com.

WebMD: This is a quick resource for a wide variety of health issues, and it brings together its own panel of physicians and health professionals and contributors, including myself. www.webmd.com.

APA report on willpower. This report provides more detail on the current state of research on willpower and self-control: apa.org/helpcenter/willpower-self-control.pdf.

Several websites on portion sizing and health guidelines are provided. These sites give general guidelines on what a portion should look like and can often provide quick tips (e.g., that a 4-ounce portion is about the size of a deck of cards). Keep in mind that none of these are intended to serve either as a substitute for medical advice or as an endorsement of all of the information provided through the websites: choosemyplate.gov.

DHHS Guidelines on Portion Sizes: hp2010.nhlbihin.net/portion/keep.htm.

NHLBI portion size changes and standards: nhlbi.nih.gov/health/public/heart/obesity/wecan/eat-right/distortion.htm.

health.gov/dietaryguidelines.

Physical Health Guidelines: health.gov/paguidelines.

Mayo Clinic Nutritional Recommendations: mayoclinic.com/health/healthy-diet/NU00200.

ADDITIONAL READING

Chapin, Andrea, and Sally Wofford-Girand. *The Honeymoon Is Over: True Stories of Love, Marriage and Divorce.* Grand Central Publishing, 2007. This is a nice collection of essays on relationships.

While I attempt to provide some guidance on using mindfulness to help you stop, slow down, and listen to your spider senses, this is not intended to be a book on mindfulness. If you want to become introduced to some mindfulness practices and a way to bring these practices into your daily life, the two titles below can get you started quite nicely.

Gunaratana, Bhante. *Mindfulness in Plain English: 20th Anniversary Edition.* Wisdom Publications 2011.

Williams, Mark, and Danny Freeman. *Mindfulness: An Eight-Week Plan for Finding Peace in a Frantic World.* Rodale Books, 2011.

This book is not intended to be job seeker's guide. I am just hoping that people consider their spider senses in all areas of their lives including work. The following classic book is published every year and does push people to look into what they want to do and consider what jobs are out there.

Bolles, Richard N. *What Color Is Your Parachute?* Ten Speed Press, 2013.

If you want to expand your repertoire in the world of humanistic and existential psychology, consider the following classics. These books have had profound personal and professional influence.

Frankl, Viktor. *Man's Search for Meaning* (1946).

May, Rollo. *Freedom and Destiny* (1981)

May, Rollo. *The Courage to Create* (1975).

May, Rollo. *Man's Search for Himself* (1969).

Rogers, Carl. *On Becoming a Person: A Therapist's View of Psychotherapy* (1961).

READING GROUP GUIDE

1. If you think about the times when you ate more—or found yourself eating mindlessly—what else was going on in your life at the time?

2. How do you feel when you throw food away? What lessons did you learn as a child about not finishing everything on your plate or wasting anything—food, clothes, stuff?

3. What do your spider senses feel like (unsettled gut, a shiver, chills)? What percentage of the time do you listen to them? Why do you ignore them?

4. What was the moment when your relationship with food or your body changed?

5. If you are currently sexually active, do you find that when you are eating mindlessly you have sex mindlessly?

6. How often do you "Are you sure" people? When is the last time you were "Are you sure-d?" Do you change your behavior as a result?

7. Do you ever find yourself going along with your stakeholders so you can "outsource blame"? How would it feel to really take responsibility for your own choices and listen to yourself?

8. How often do you find yourself defending your toxic stakeholders? Or a stakeholder that leads you to silence your spider senses? Why do you think that is?

9. Where do your big ticket fears come from? How long have they been with you? Have you ever faced a fear head-on? What happened? Would you do it again?

10. Has there ever been a time when you made a decision against your best interests or defied good sense (gatekeeping) because you thought "It will be different for me"? In which areas of your life do you find it most difficult to gatekeep? Food? Work? Relationships?

11. What sources of data do you go to most frequently (e.g. Internet, people)? Do these sources of data work in line with your spider

senses or throw them off? What sorts of data do you find difficult to rely on? Are there people in your life whose data or advice you find yourself reliant on? And conversely, are there people in your life whose data or advice you find problematic?

12. Think about the Promise of One "backwards." In other words, reflect on a time when you did do something you wanted—built a room on your house, finished a degree, started a club—and think about how you got there. Was it a few things each day over a period of time? The Promise of One gets some of its power when you think about the fact that you may already be doing it and not even realizing it.

13. Do you think there are some people you will never learn to be able to eat well around?

14. What are the biggest daily stressors in your life? Do you see the connection between those daily stressors and how your willpower gets depleted?

15. Have you ever attempted meditation or other mindfulness practices? Did you enjoy them? Find them problematic? What makes meditation or mindfulness difficult for you?

16. How often do you use trigger foods to manage emotional states (broken hearts, bad day at work, fight with a friend)? How do you manage trigger foods now? Is it working? How did they become trigger foods?

17. For you personally, what are the connections between food and life? How do your eating patterns vary with your relationships? Family life? Work? Do you eat more or less when you are happy? Sad? Frustrated? Angry? Stressed?

18. Do you find that the mistakes you make at work (for example being unwilling to change jobs even though you are miserable) are similar to the mistakes you make at the table (for example, being unable to say no to seconds)?

19. If you were to choose an area of your life that you think is most in need of an overhaul (relationships, family life, finances, work, other areas), what would it be?

20. Do you see the connection between your relationship life and your eating life? Are there parallels in the patterns? What are the glues that bind the intimate relationship you are in (or if you are not in a relationship, the relationships you have been in)? Connection? Culture? Stakeholders? Scripts? Love? Fear? Other things?

21. How is your committed/intimate relationship (or lack of a relationship) contributing to your struggles with weight and eating?

22. How do you feel after you shop? Do you enjoy shopping? Do you use it as a way to fill emptiness? Does shopping co-exist with other regulation problems? For example, do you go shopping and find yourself eating out on those days and eating more than you intended?

23. If you were to make big changes in your life, who are you the most afraid of losing? What would happen if you lost him or her?

24. Can you think of examples of trying to buy "insurance" for life to avoid things like a broken heart? Is it possible that you maintain your weight as a way to keep scary experiences like relationships, shifts at work, and taking on your dreams at a distance?

25. What do you want your life to look like? What are the barriers that hold you back from living authentically?

INDEX

ABOUT THE AUTHOR

Dr. Ramani Durvasula is a co-host and psychologist on *My Shopping Addiction,* a new series on Oxygen Network, and she was featured on Bravo's *THINtervention.* Her talk- and news-show appearances include *Dr. Oz, Dr. Drew's Lifechangers,* and *Anderson Cooper.* She is a professor of psychology at California State University, Los Angeles, and a licensed clinical psychologist. She lives in Los Angeles. Visit her at doctor-ramani.com.

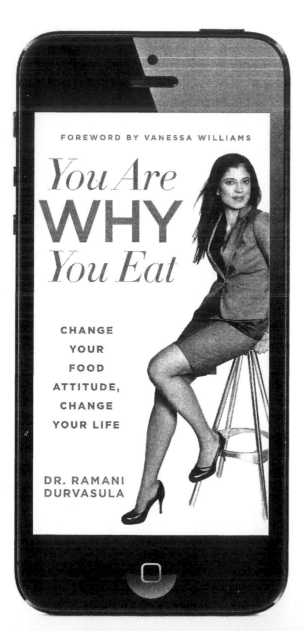
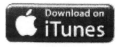